OXFORD MEDICAL PUBLICATIONS

DENTAL RADIOLOGY

Dental Radiology

Understanding the X-ray Image

●

LAETITIA BROCKLEBANK

Senior Lecturer in Oral Radiology
University of Glasgow

and

Honorary Consultant in Oral Radiology
Greater Glasgow Health Board
formerly
Lecturer in Oral Radiology
University of Hong Kong

Oxford   New York   Tokyo
OXFORD UNIVERSITY PRESS
1997

Oxford University Press, Great Clarendon Street, Oxford OX2 6DP

Oxford   New York

Athens   Auckland   Bangkok   Bogota   Bombay   Buenos Aires
Calcutta   Cape Town   Dar es Salaam   Delhi   Florence   Hong Kong
Istanbul   Karachi   Kuala Lumpur   Madras   Madrid   Melbourne
Mexico City   Nairobi   Paris   Singapore   Taipei   Tokyo   Toronto
and associated companies in
Berlin   Ibadan

Oxford is a trade mark of Oxford University Press

Published in the United States
by Oxford University Press Inc., New York

A catalogue record for this book is available from the British Library

Library of Congress Cataloging-in-Publication Data
Brocklebank, Laetitia.
Dental radiology: understanding the X-ray image / Laetitia Brocklebank.
(Oxford medical publications)
Includes bibliographical references and index.
1. Teeth — Radiology. 2. Teeth — Diseases — Diagnosis.
I. Title. II. Series.
[DNLM: 1. Radiology, Dental. 2. Tooth — radiology. WN 230
B864d   1996]
RK309.875   1996   617.6′07572 — dc20   96–47906
ISBN 0–19–262410–5 (pbk). — ISBN 0–19–262411–3 (Hbk)

Typeset by EXPO Holdings, Malaysia
Printed in Great Britain by The Bath Press

Preface

This book on understanding dental radiology has developed from my experience of discussing radiographic images with dental practitioners and students. There are a number of textbooks available on dental and maxillo-facial radiology, which are usually targeted at the undergraduate, or specializing postgraduate. Many of these are excellent texts, but they are not intended primarily to meet the requirements of the practising dentist. This book is designed for that purpose, to provide clear, practical information for the practitioner, supported by checklists, and numerous illustrations, to assist in resolving areas of difficulty in radiological diagnosis.

My objective is to illustrate the variety of radiographic images of the teeth and their supporting structures, according to anatomical location, or their key descriptive feature. The radiographs have been chosen to illustrate a logical approach to interpreting the images, to help in gleaning as much information as possible about the conditions affecting the patient's teeth, in order to assist and support in their diagnosis and treatment.

The sequence of the chapters is designed to reflect the approach to examination of radiographs that forms the basis of the book, which is described fully in Chapter 3. The first four chapters are core material which will enhance the subsequent, more descriptive chapters. The remaining chapters are designed so that they can be read alone, and in any order, if required.

This book is intended to appeal to the reader who has an enquiring mind, some existing knowledge of dentistry, and a desire to enhance their understanding of the radiographic images that they see routinely, and those that they only encounter occasionally.

July 1996   Laetitia Brocklebank
Glasgow

Acknowledgements

No book on radiology would be possible without the skilled expertise of the radiographers responsible for the images, and all the other personnel who support this process. I have been fortunate to work in a number of dental teaching hospitals, and been able to build up a collection of material for teaching purposes. The majority of material used in this book has come from my time at the Prince Philip Dental Hospital in Hong Kong; the Edinburgh Dental Hospital; and the Glasgow Dental Hospital & School, where I had the opportunity to work with many excellent radiographers. I would like to record especially the Superintendents of each department: Dennis Brown (Tutor at PPDH), Maggie Phillips (EDH), and Helen Shanks and Marysia Wylupek (GDH&S). In addition my special thanks to Professor David Smith and Mr Eric Whaites for permission to use a few radiographs from their collections at King's College Hospital and Guy's Hospital; and to colleagues for enabling me to produce the following illustrations: Helen Milne (Fig. 4.9 and Fig. 4.10) and Glenn Frew (Fig. D1). Figures 4.4b and 8.24 have been reproduced here with kind permission of the publishers Churchill Livingstone, and Butterworth-Heinemann, for which grateful acknowledgements.

Many people have supported me in this venture, not least everyone who has worked with me over the last few years at Glasgow, and whose hard work enabled me to devote time to this project. They cannot all be mentioned by name, as any attempt to do so would inevitably result in omissions. My acknowledgements to all the staff in the various Radiology departments: radiographers, darkroom, secretarial, and reception staff — they have each played a part in building up this collection. I appreciate that without the clinicians who refer the patients none of the material would exist. The staff of the departments of Dental Illustration have provided invaluable support in reproduction of many of the images, especially the photographic images produced for this project.

I would like to take this opportunity to thank by name just four people, without whom this book would not have come to fruition: Professor David Smith with whom I studied for an M.Sc. He inspired my love of dental radiology, and freely gave me advice in the early stages of this project — other students of his will perhaps recognise some of him in my writing; Julie Hoare of OUP who patiently discussed this book with me over a number of years, and became a good friend in the process; Dr Alan Campbell for his generous advice, and without whom I would perhaps never have studied dentistry; and finally, to my husband, Malcolm, especial thanks for his unwavering support and belief in me.

To everyone who has supported and helped me with this book thank you very much.

1996   Laetitia Brocklebank

Foreword

Professor N. J. D. Smith
King's Dental Institute
London

As the end of an academic career comes closer, one of the great pleasures that comes is in watching the blossoming careers of young men and women first known as young students.

This is especially true of Laetitia Brocklebank, who first came to my department as a postgraduate student in 1977. During the intervening years Laetitia has amassed a wealth of experience, first heading the Unit of Oral Radiology in the recently opened Prince Philip Dental Hospital in Hong Kong, where she had to build up a teaching programme from scratch; then a period at the Edinburgh Dental School and now at the Glasgow Dental School. This experience is encapsulated in *Dental Radiology*.

There is a growing number of comprehensive and very expensive text books on dental and maxillofacial radiology which are available to the specialist. Laetitia Brocklebank has correctly identified the need for a rather shorter and more practical volume which will, in her own words, be written for the general practitioner. I think that she is, perhaps, being unduly modest and that this book will be equally useful for the dental undergraduate who is approaching his or her final examinations.

The approach is essentially practical. When confronted with a radiograph, the practitioner is more often than not able to recognize that something is amiss and so this book is essentially structured round the anatomical regions involved. This is, in many ways, a more logical way of looking at abnormality than the conventional classification of disease entities.

Of course, these two approaches are not mutually exclusive, but I suspect that the practitioner in his surgery would find it easier to use the approach adopted here.

Although I am sure this excellent book will also be found in Dental School Libraries, its place is in the dental surgery near the viewing box.

CONTENTS

1 PRODUCTION OF RADIOGRAPHS   1

   1.1 Introduction   2
   1.2 The radiographic image   2
   1.3 Production of a radiograph   2

2 RADIOGRAPHIC PROJECTIONS AND ANATOMICAL FEATURES   17

   2.1 Introduction   18
   2.2 Radiographic projections   18
   2.3 Lists of anatomical features   31

3 EXAMINATION OF RADIOGRAPHS   43

   3.1 Introduction   44
   3.2 Checklist   45
   3.3 Details of components of checklist   46
   3.4 Applications   67

4 LOCALIZATION USING DENTAL RADIOGRAPHY   69

   4.1 Introduction   70
   4.2 Viewing radiographs   71
   4.3 Views at right-angles   72
   4.4 Parallax   74
   4.5 Useful radiographic combinations   80
   4.6 Poor combinations   85
   4.7 Radiopaque markers   86
   4.8 Self-assessment examples   87
   4.9 Answers to self-assessment examples   87

5 CORONAL AND PERICORONAL CHANGES   93

   5.1 Introduction   94
   5.2 Normal appearance and developmental changes   94
   5.3 Abnormalities   95

6 PULP AND ROOT CHANGES   107

   6.1 Introduction   108
   6.2 Normal structure and development   108
   6.3 Abnormalities   110
   6.4 Short roots   116

7 BONE: PERIAPICAL AND PERIODONTAL 121
7.1 Introduction 122
7.2 Normal periodontal and periapical structures 122
7.3 Inflammatory changes 126
7.4 Non-inflammatory pathological periapical changes 133

8 RADIOLUCENT LESIONS 137
8.1 Introduction 138
8.2 Sites and materials involved 138
8.3 Radiolucencies 138

9 RADIOPAQUE AND COMBINATION LESIONS 159
9.1 Introduction 160
9.2 Sites and materials involved 160
9.3 Radiopaque and combination lesions 160

10 DENTAL TRAUMA 175
10.1 Introduction 176
10.2 Causes of dental trauma 176
10.3 Radiography 182
10.4 Radiological appearance 183

Appendix A: Key components in the dental X-ray tube: checklist 184

Appendix B: Lists of anatomical features 186

Appendix C: Examination of radiographs: checklist 190

Appendix D: Specialized imaging techniques 192
            D.1 Ionizing radiation 192
            D.2 Non-ionizing radiation 205

BIBLIOGRAPHY 209

INDEX 211

1 Production of radiographs

1.1   INTRODUCTION   2
1.2   THE RADIOGRAPHIC IMAGE   2
1.3   PRODUCTION OF A RADIOGRAPH   2

1.3.1 The source of X-rays   3
1.3.2 Interaction of X-rays with matter   7
1.3.3 The object   9
1.3.4 Image receptors   10
1.3.5 Processing   14
1.3.6 Mounting and storage systems   15
1.3.7 Viewing systems   15

1   Production of radiographs

1.1   INTRODUCTION

Radiological interpretation is dependent on the ability to make observations and to interpret them within a framework of knowledge. An awareness of how the radiographic image is produced, and the key factors that influence the image, is a necessary component of the knowledge base. This chapter will review the key aspects of radiographic image production, and is supported by a checklist of facts in Appendix A.

1.2   THE RADIOGRAPHIC IMAGE

Radiographs are two-dimensional images generated by the interaction of X-rays and tissues, which depict variations in the types and nature of structures (influenced by atomic number, density, and thickness), permanently recorded in emulsion that is supported by a plastic base. The first part of this statement is fact: as a complete statement, its truth is dependent on a series of procedures being carried out correctly.

1.   Suitable exposure factors are necessary to result in an appropriate pattern of X-ray energies in the beam after passing through the object, in order to sensitize the film emulsion and create a latent image.

2.   Processing procedures must be correctly carried out in order to make the 'latent image' in the emulsion permanently visible and non-degradable.

3.   Storage systems must be adequate to ensure retrieval of images when required.

These three points relate particularly to images on radiographic film, which is the method used for the majority of dental radiographs. It is also possible to produce images using electrostatically charged plates and, more recently, computer systems in conjunction with a source of X-rays; the use of direct digital radiography is increasing, and brief notes are provided in Appendix D. The interpretation of the final image is facilitated by the system proposed in this book, which is largely independent of the precise method of production of the image.

1.3   PRODUCTION OF A RADIOGRAPH

In order to produce and use a radiograph it is necessary to have:

(1)   a source of X-rays;

(2)   interaction between X-rays and the object matter;

(3)   an object requiring X-ray examination;

(4)   an appropriate image receptor;

(5)   a processing system;

(6)   a storage system;

(7)   a viewing system.

These seven areas will be looked at in turn in order to provide a practical scientific background to the production of radiographic images of the dental and maxillo-facial region.

1.3.1   The source of X-rays

X-rays are a form of electromagnetic radiation as are light and radio waves, and are similar in their potential actions to naturally occurring gamma-rays. X-rays are man-made and produced by interactions which occur within atoms of certain materials when fast-moving electrons are rapidly decelerated by collision with that material. The general properties of X-rays are similar to all electromagnetic radiations: they travel in straight lines and diverge from a point source, obeying the *inverse square law* (Box 1.1). They also have unique

---

Box 1.1

The inverse square law states that the intensity of a beam of electromagnetic radiation is inversely proportional to the square of the distance from the origin.

---

properties which result in their use in imaging (Box 1.2). Unfortunately, the same mechanisms that are useful in image production, are capable of causing physical and biological damage, such that their use must be carefully controlled.

Box 1.2

Properties of X-rays
- Travel in straight lines
- Obey inverse square law
- Cause certain elements to fluoresce
- Interact with certain photographic emulsions
- Interact with matter, according to atomic number of elements, and energy value of X-rays
- Not detectable by human senses

The components of a typical dental X-ray tube provide a useful basis for understanding the production of X-rays. Appendix A contains brief factual notes on the properties of these components. The function of each is discussed in greater detail in this section and their position is illustrated in the diagrammatic representation of a dental X-ray tube in Fig. 1.1. A number of features concerning the operation of an X-ray tube are controlled in the United Kingdom by the Ionising Radiations Regulations[1]; the regulations pertinent to dental radiography are reproduced in a handbook: *Radiation protection in dental practice*. The important points in the regulations that refer to various aspects of the X-ray tube will be reproduced where relevant.

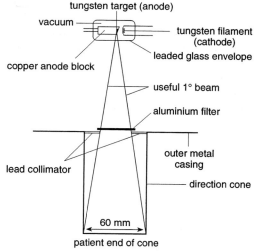

Fig. 1.1   Diagrammatic representation of dental X-ray tube key components (not to scale).

Cathode

A tungsten filament, forming the negative pole of the X-ray tube. It is heated by passing a small current (7–15 mA) through it, resulting in electrons being released from the atoms and forming a cloud around the filament, similar to steam over boiling water. Tungsten has a high melting point (3410 °C) which prevents it from disintegrating in spite of the intense heat generated by the current. Due to its high atomic number (Z = 74) it is an efficient producer of relatively large numbers of electrons when treated in this way.

Anode

A small block of tungsten (the target), forming the positive pole of the X-ray tube, set into a larger copper block at an angle of approximately 20° to a line parallel to the cathode filament. The resulting effective focal spot size is usually 0.7 mm². It is in this small tungsten target that interactions occur between the electrons generated at the cathode and the electrons and nuclei of the tungsten atoms, resulting in X-ray production. The cathode electrons are made to bombard the target at high speed by applying a potential difference between the cathode and the anode, the cathode being negative and the anode positive, with respect to each other. The potential difference in dental X-ray tubes is in the order of 50–100 kV (kilovolts); the recommended optimum kV for dental radiography is 60–70 kV (see *Guidelines on Radiology & Standards* 1994[2]). This high voltage is achieved by a step-up transformer incorporated within the dental X-ray set and supplied from a normal domestic power supply.

Anode block

The large copper block surrounding the tungsten target provides an efficient method of conducting heat away from the target. Over 99 per cent of the interactions between the bombarding electrons and the tungsten atoms result in heat production and this needs to be removed as rapidly as possible in order to enable the next X-ray exposure to be made, and to prolong the working life of the tube.

Reinforced glass surround

The cathode and anode are contained in a glass envelope which is reinforced in order to enable all the air to be evacuated from inside. It is necessary for the electrons to pass through a vacuum as they would otherwise become involved in interactions with air molecules, effectively reducing the efficiency of the system still further.

Lead shielding and tube housing

The X-ray tube head incorporates lead in order to prevent X-rays leaking out of the tube (Box 1.3). Only those to be directed at the object under inves-

---

Box 1.3

Leakage radiation: every X-ray source assembly (comprising an X-ray tube, an X-ray tube housing, and a beam limiting device) should be constructed so that, at every rating specified by the manufacturer for that X-ray source assembly, the air kerma from the leakage radiation at a distance from the focal-spot of 1 m averaged over an area not exceeding 100 cm² does not exceed 1 mGy* in one hour.

---

*mGy = milliGray

tigation are intentionally allowed to leave through a defined 'window' in the shielding. Lead is an extremely efficient absorber of X-rays due to its high atomic number (Z = 82).

Window

There is a small opening in the lead casing through which the X-ray beam is directed. This is referred to as the window and is located directly under the external direction indicating device commonly referred to as the 'cone'. The useful X-ray beam (the primary beam) exits from the tube through the window. The beam diverges from its point of origin, until it is stopped by reactions with matter, and obeying the inverse square law it decreases in intensity with increasing distance from the source.

Collimator

The collimator is the part that controls the shape and size of the beam (Box 1.4); it is made of lead and the resultant shape of the X-ray beam is either circular or rectangular; the rectangular shape introduced in the newest machines matches the shape of the intra-oral X-ray film packets, and results in a considerable reduction in X-ray dose to the patient. The collimator is either permanently located in the tube head or at the tube head end of the removable directional cone; a universal rectangular collimator is available to fit into the patient end of circular cones.

Box 1.4

Beam diameter : the beam diameter should not exceed 60 mm measured at the patient end of the cone.

Cone

All X-ray tubes are fitted with some method of directing the beam at the patient. In dental X-ray machines this is normally in the form of a removable direction indicating device which may be cylindrical or rectangular in form. Older machines still in use may have pointed cones, and the descriptive word 'cone' is still traditionally used, regardless of the actual shape. Some cylindrical cones are lined with lead in order to continue to define the sharp cut-off of the beam, thus providing secondary collimation. Plastic cylindrical directional cones have no direct influence on the shape or area of the X-ray beam.

The cone determines the minimum distance between the X-ray source and the patient's skin (Box 1.5).

Box 1.5

Distance control : field defining spacer cones should ensure a focal-spot to skin distance of not less than 200 mm (20 cm) for equipment operating above 60 kV and not less than 100 mm (10 cm) for equipment operating at lower voltages.

Oil

The glass envelope is surrounded by oil which fulfils two functions: (1) to act as an insulator and reduce the risk of electrical problems; (2) to act as a secondary method of heat distribution, oil being an efficient conductor of heat.

Aluminum filter

There is a need to remove the low-energy X-rays from the beam before they reach the patient, where they will add to the patient dose by interacting with the soft tissues, without the benefit of providing useful information in the final image. These X-rays arise from the electron–nucleus interactions in the target, and need to be filtered out. Aluminum is an efficient absorber of low-energy X-rays, in the region of 2 keV, which are not useful for image production, but would add to the patient's absorbed dose. Minimum thicknesses are specified (Box 1.6).

Box 1.6

Beam filtration : the total filtration of the beam should be equivalent to not less than:
(a)   1.5 mm aluminum for voltages up to and including 70 kV.
(b)   2.5 mm aluminium (of which 1.5 mm is permanent) for voltages above 70 kV.

Target interactions

The target, or anode, of the X-ray tube is the site of production of X-rays. The incoming electrons interact with the tungsten atoms in two important ways resulting in a transfer of energy and a change in the form of the energy.

1.   Electron–nucleus interactions.

2.   Electron–electron interactions.

The concepts important to these interactions in the target, and those between X-rays and matter, require an understanding of the basic structure of an atom (Box 1.7).

Box 1.7

Conceptual structure of an atom
A nucleus, containing protons (positively charged) and neutrons (no charge), is surrounded by orbiting electrons (negative charge). The orbits are referred to by letters, K,L,M,N,O, etc., with K being nearest the nucleus. The maximum number of electrons possible in an orbit is mathematically related to the orbit in numeral terms, K being referred to as 1, M as 3, etc.
Maximum possible number of electrons = $n^2 \times 2$, where n = the orbit number, e.g.
K orbit, $n = 1$, $n^2 = 1$, $\times\ 2 = 2$
M orbit, $n = 3$, $n^2 = 9$, $\times\ 2 = 18$, giving the following potential numbers of electrons: K = 2, L = 8, M = 18, N = 32, O = 50.
Two numbers are important in relation to atoms:
Z, the atomic number is equal to the number of electrons, which equals the number of protons in a stable atom.
A, the atomic mass number is equal to the sum of the number of protons and neutrons.

---

1. Electron–nucleus interactions

An electron passing close to the nucleus of an atom will come under the influence of the nucleus, which exerts a powerful force on the electron, causing it to slow down and alter its direction of travel, having released some of its energy. The majority of the energy (approximately 99 per cent) is released as heat, which is of no value to the diagnostic process and needs to be removed as rapidly as possible in order not to cause damage to the target from overheating. A very small proportion of the energy (less than 1 per cent) is in the form of X-ray photons. The X-ray photons produced in this way are often referred to as 'Bremsstrahlung' radiation (the German word for 'braking'), as this graphically explains how they are produced. These X-ray photons have energy levels covering the whole range of kilovoltages up to the applied voltage. The spectrum of energy levels explains another commonly used name for this type of X-ray beam of 'white radiation', in the same way as white light comprises the whole spectrum of individual colours.

2. Electron–electron interactions

A proportion of the electrons in the stream directed at the target may have energy levels greater than that of some of the binding energies of the electrons in the target atoms; the possibility of this occurring is dependent on both the target material and the applied kilovoltage. With a tungsten target this will only occur with applied voltages of greater than 69 kVp*.

An incoming electron that passes close to a bound electron is able to eject it from its orbit if its energy level is greater than the value of the binding energy. The atom is now in an unstable state, and returns to stability by filling the vacancy from outer orbits and ultimately attracting a free electron. At each stage of this electron transfer energy is released, according to the difference in the binding energies of the two orbits; the value of this energy in electron volts is characteristic to each element, and to the electron shells involved. Tungsten is capable of producing characteristic radiation in this way with energy levels that are within the X-ray section of electromagnetic radiation, of approximately 58 and 68 keV.

The X-rays produced in the target are multi-directional, and their exit from the tube, and direction are therefore controlled by the tube housing and the collimator.

1.3.2 Interaction of X-rays with matter

There are four possible fates for an X-ray photon passing through matter, when considering dental radiography:

1. The X-rays can pass straight through without modification.
2. The X-rays can be completely absorbed by the material.
3. The X-rays can be scattered, and change their direction of travel, losing energy at the same time.
4. The X-rays can be scattered, and change their direction of travel, without losing energy.

*kVp = peak kilovoltage (maximum applied voltage).

The processes of *absorption* and *scatter* together result in *attenuation* of the X-ray beam, which is a variable reduction in intensity of the beam. Absorption is both useful and potentially damaging, whereas scatter has no advantages and is potentially damaging to the image, the patient, and any other persons in the immediate vicinity of the X-ray tube. The mechanisms by which these two processes occur, and the factors which most strongly influence them are covered in this section.

Photoelectric absorption

The process resulting in absorption of an X-ray photon is termed 'photoelectric absorption' as it is based on a two-part interaction: first, the photon energy is absorbed; and secondly, characteristic radiation is released according to the electron binding energies of the element involved in the interaction.

This occurs sequentially in the following stages:

(1) an incoming X-ray photon passes very close to a bound electron in an inner orbital shell;

(2) if the X-ray photon has energy just greater than the binding energy of the electron then the electron will be ejected from its shell, and from the atom; this electron is then free to be captured by another atom, and is no longer of relevance to this particular interaction;

(3) the atom is now in an unstable state and in order to return to stability needs to fill the vacancy in the inner orbit. This occurs by an electron from the next outer, or next but one outer shell dropping in to fill the vacancy. There are differences in the binding energies of the successive shells, and the difference in binding energies is released as characteristic radiation. The characteristic radiation will be in the form of one of the electromagnetic radiations, according to its energy value, measured in electron volts. Only relatively high-energy radiations are of interest in their potential for further interactions;

(4) the vacant outer positions in the outer orbital shells are successively filled, with the capture of a free electron allowing the atom to return to stability.

It will be clear that this process is essentially the same as the production of characteristic radiation in the anode of the X-ray tube.

The probability of photoelectric absorption occurring is strongly dependent on the atomic number (Z) of the material involved, and the peak kilovoltage of the X-ray beam; in each case the probability is related to the cube of the factor.

Probability $\propto Z^3$
Probability inversely $\propto kV^3$

A list of atomic numbers relevant to dentistry is included in Appendix A; reference to this will explain why lead, with an atomic number of 82, is such a good absorber of X-rays, whereas soft tissue with an effective atomic number of 7 is a rather poor absorber. The actual difference in atomic numbers, between natural tissues in the body, is very little; the cubed values adopt a greater level of significance.

Soft tissue $Z = 7$ $Z^3 =$ 343
Bone $Z = 12$ $Z^3 = 1728$

Scatter

Scattering can occur in two ways:

(1)   unmodified (synonyms: elastic, Raleigh)

(2)   modified (synonyms: inelastic, Compton)

The second type, most commonly referred to as Compton scatter, is of most interest in diagnostic radiography, and is a combination of absorption and redistribution of energy. It occurs more frequently with photons of greater energy than those predominantly involved in the photoelectric absorption effect.

The probability of Compton scattering occurring is not dependent on atomic number in the same way as photoelectric absorption, but is dependent on electron density, which can vary within a single material according to its state (e.g. water has a greater electron density than steam although both consist of H_2O). It will inevitably tend to occur to a greater extent in atoms having a higher atomic number, due to their relatively greater number of electrons.

The process commences in the same way as photoelectric absorption, but at the point of ejection of the bound electron there exists an excess of photon energy; this energy is re-released as a scatter, or secondary, X-ray photon of lower energy than the original photon.

scatter energy = original photon energy – binding energy of ejected electron

In addition to the energy value changing considerably the scatter photon changes its direction of travel. Every scatter photon produced is then able to undergo a further interaction, and ultimately the energy will be completely absorbed by the material concerned.

1.3.3   The object

In dental radiography the objects of primary interest are the teeth and jaws and in some situations the related soft tissue structures. These provide a natural variety of tissue types (e.g. enamel, dentine, and various connective tissues), and within some tissue types a variation of structural form (e.g. bone may be cancellous or cortical according to the trabecular arrangement). The normal appearance of anatomical features in a variety of X-ray projections is discussed in Chapter 2.

It is the differences between structures or within a structure that result in a recognizable radiographic image, following interaction between X-rays and the component atoms.

The appearance of everyday objects can be helpful in understanding how different materials, and the particular perspective from which they are viewed, can influence the image that is observed; these observations can then be applied to images of the teeth and jaws.

Thin, symmetrical objects, with no internal structural variation, have similarities in their visual and radiographic appearances. In both types of image there is sharp definition of their margins (Figs 1.2 and 1.3).

Objects with considerable depth often look quite different when viewed from different vantage points, as different aspects are presented to the eye. As X-rays have the potential to partially pass through many materials, it is reasonable to expect that there will be less difference in X-ray images; the image will, however, be influenced by which particular facet of the object is closest to the image receptor, due to the divergent nature of the X-ray beam. An egg

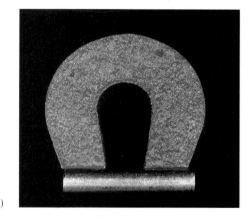

(a)

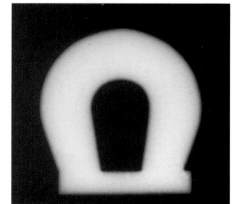

(b)

Fig. 1.2
(a) An iron magnet.
(b) X-ray image.

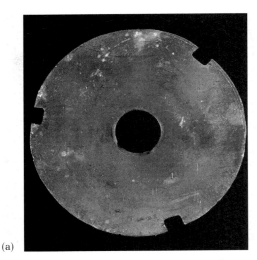

(a)

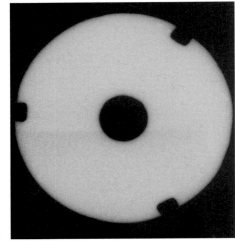

(b)

Fig. 1.3   (a) A lead disc. b) X-ray image.

cup and ramekin dish, as seen from three different vantage points visually and radiographically (Figs 1.4–1.7), illustrate this point.

There are a number of interesting points to be observed from this series of images.

1. In the *visual images* there is no information about surfaces of the object that are not facing the observer, or about the internal construction of the object.

2. These *radiograpic images* illustrate how the relationship of the object to the film, combined with the divergence of the X-ray beam, influences the resultant image:

    (a) when the objects are in their normal upright position, with the base closest to the X-ray film (Figs 1.5a and 1.7a), the upper rim, which has the largest circumference, is projected outside the images of the edges and the base by the divergence of the X-ray beam; the ridged wall of the ramekin dish is clearly depicted;

    (b) when the object is turned upside down (as in Figs 1.4b and 1.6b), so that the rim is closest to the film (Figs 1.5b and 1.7b), the smaller base is projected further out, and becomes superimposed on the larger rim; the ridges of the ramekin dish are also superimposed and no longer clearly depicted; the external facets of the egg cup are however clearer in this image, as they are projected beyond the rim.

3. In both the egg cup and the ramekin dish, clear, thin white lines are seen in the profile radiographs (Figs 1.5c and 1.7c), representing the inner surfaces of the objects, and specific portions of the external surfaces; the difference between the two is that the external aspect of the ridges of the ramekin dish is depicted, but not the external aspect of the egg cup: in the egg cup the X-ray beam passes at a tangent to the outer circumference, whereas in the ramekin dish it passes through a complete ridge which presents sufficient depth of material to the beam to affect its attenuation.

4. The X-ray image is sensitive enough to demonstrate quite subtle variations in thickness of a material that absorbs X-rays. The printing on the base of the ramekin dish is painted on the surface and readily visible in Fig. 1.6b, but has no effect on the X-ray image. In contrast, the lettering on the base of the egg cup is part of the construction of the object and has no distinguishing colour to make it clearly visible in the photograph; in the radiograph (Fig. 1.5d) the pattern can be detected on the base due to varying attenuation.

1.3.4   Image receptors

The image receptors most commonly used in dental radiography are conventional intra-oral film, directly sensitive to X-ray photons, and screen–film combinations in extra-oral cassettes, where the intensifying screens are sensitive to X-ray photons and the film is sensitive to light of specific wavelengths.

Intra-oral X-ray film

The intra-oral film packet contains film emulsion which is directly sensitive to the X-ray wavelengths used in dental radiography. The components of a typical intra-oral film packet are shown in Fig. 1.8, and the function of each part is summarized below.

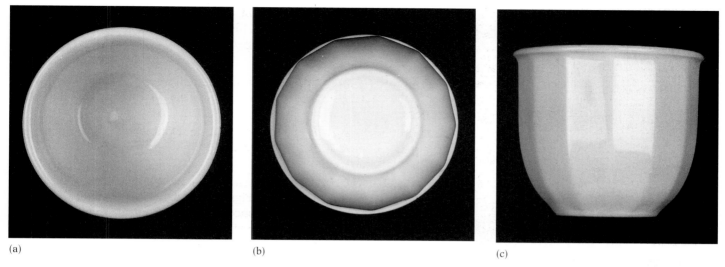

(a)   (b)   (c)

Fig. 1.4   Three different views of an egg cup.   (a) Looking into it from above.   (b) Looking at the base.   (c) Side view.

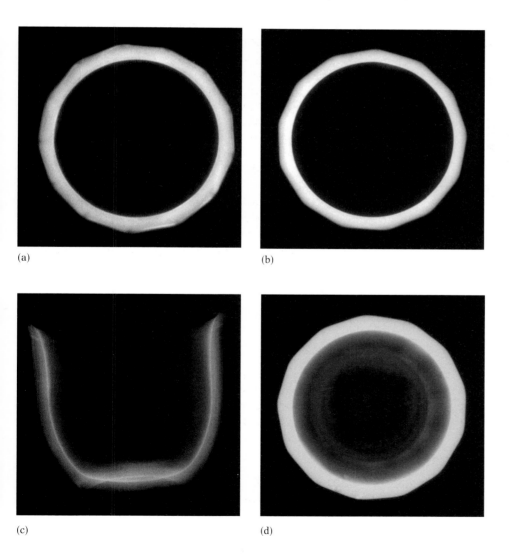

(a)   (b)

(c)   (d)

Fig. 1.5   Four different radiographic projections of the egg cup.
(a) The base is closest to the film.
(b) The upper rim is closest to the film.
(c) Side view.
(d) Base view, reduced exposure.

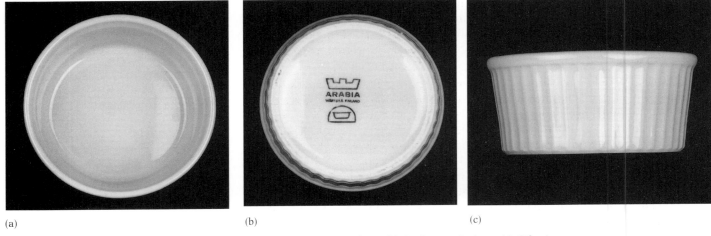

(a)   (b)   (c)

Fig. 1.6   Three different views of a ramekin dish. (a) Looking into it from above. (b) Looking at the base. (c) Side view.

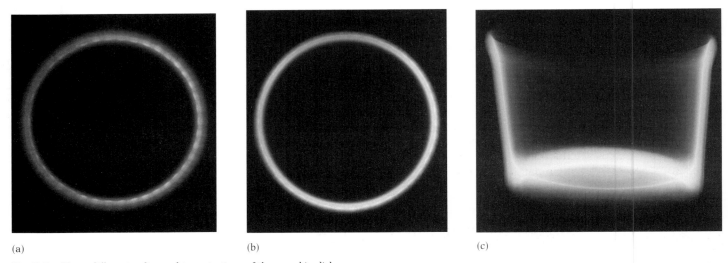

(a)   (b)   (c)

Fig. 1.7   Three different radiographic projections of the ramekin dish.
(a) The base is closest to the film.   (b) The upper rim is closest to the film.   (c) Side view.

1. *Outer covering.* This is either plastic or reinforced paper. It serves the purpose of preventing moisture in the oral cavity reaching the sensitive emulsion, and also acts as a light barrier. The tube side is usually plain in colour; the colour on the reverse indicates film speed. Most manufacturers include written information about the film type.

2. *Dark inner paper lining.* This has two main functions: (1) to act as a secondary barrier to light should there be any breach in the outer covering, too small to be seen visually but large enough to result in deterioration of the film due to light exposure; (2) incorporation of a small flap at the open end of the film packet by some manufacturers assists in easy removal of the film from the packet when processing is carried out after exposure to X-rays.

3. *X-ray film.* The film used for dental radiography consists of a plastic base with emulsion on both sides. The active constituent of the emulsion is predominantly silver bromide and will respond to light as well as X-ray

wavelengths. The plastic base to the emulsion provides rigidity when the film is still in its packaging and also later when it becomes a radiograph which can be viewed by transmitted light. Manufacturers normally add a tint to the plastic base in order to make the image more acceptable to the human eye.

4.   *Lead foil.* A piece of thin lead foil which normally incorporates an embossed pattern is positioned inside the film packet on the non-tube side of the film. As already noted, lead is a very efficient absorber of X-rays. It is incorporated in the film packet in order to absorb any X-rays which are directed at the film other than through the object of interest; X-rays approaching the film from other directions will result in a general fogging of the image, making it less clear and therefore less easy to interpret. The embossed pattern on the lead foil is a safety feature so that if a radiograph is taken with the film packet positioned back to front the foil pattern enables recognition of the precise fault; although an image will still be produced, it will be a lighter image, and it is important not to confuse this fault with under-exposure.

5.   *Embossed dot.* All components of the intra-oral film packet are embossed with a raised dot near one corner*. The convex aspect of the dot is directed towards the X-ray tube. This feature enables the film packet to be properly positioned in the mouth, and the processed radiograph to be viewed correctly.

Extra-oral film and intensifying screens

The use of intensifying screens, which produce visible light as a result of photoelectric interactions between X-ray photons and the active components of the screen, enables a reduction in X-ray exposure to be achieved. There is some loss of resolution as compared to direct film images and this, together

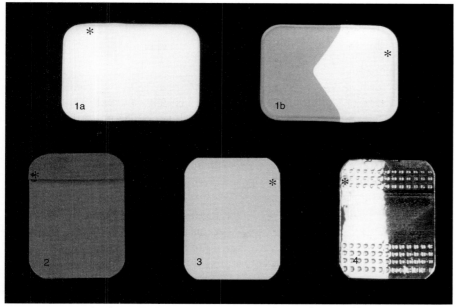

1a. outer covering front 1b. outer covering back 2. dark paper lining 3. *X*-ray film 4. lead foil

Fig. 1.8 Intra-oral film packet and component parts.

with the unavoidable bulk, makes such a combination impractical for routine intra-oral radiography. Intensifying screen–film combinations are used for panoramic radiography and all other extra-oral radiographic techniques. An extra-oral cassette opened to show the intensifying screens is shown in Fig. 1.9.

There are two main groups of screens available, each characterized by different coloured light emissions, which must be used in conjunction with film sensitive to that colour. Common materials and their light emissions are listed in Box 1.8.

> **Box 1.8**
>
> *Intensifying screen: colour emission*
> 1. Calcium tungstate: blue light.
> 2. Rare earth materials, such as those from the lanthanum and gadolinium series: green light.

Intensifying screen interactions

These screens utilize the property of X-rays that causes certain materials to fluoresce, as a result of photoelectric interactions. The light produced is used to expose light-sensitive film, and the inherent efficiency of the system allows a considerable reduction in radiation exposure, when compared to the equivalent dose received from a direct film examination. Fluorescence is the instantaneous emission of light, with no afterglow, as opposed to phosphorescence where there is a glow of some duration after the main event. Glow-worms are a good example of phosphorescence, and exhibit a slow release of the energy captured in surface cells.

Calcium tungstate was previously the traditional material used for intensifying screens. In recent years, however, a number of rare earth materials have been utilized as they are more efficient at producing light and therefore reduce the radiation exposure even further. The most frequently used rare earth materials are from the Gadolinium and Lanthanum series of elements. The term 'rare' is due to the difficulty in separating them from the other elements with which they are naturally found.

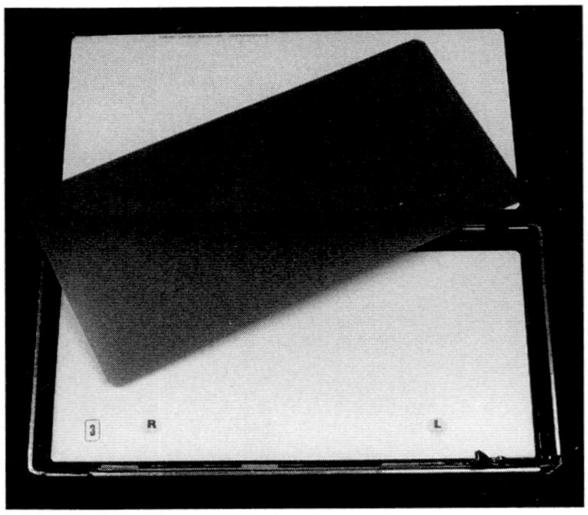

Emulsion interactions

The atomic level interactions of X-ray photons with the silver bromide crystals in the emulsion of both intra-oral and extra-oral film are very similar to the interactions that occur between X-ray photons and atoms within the body or other materials placed in the path of the X-ray beam; these are also similar to the interactions occurring between the electrons and the target atoms within the anode of the X-ray tube.

The interactions that occur in the emulsion result in a latent image formed by the pattern of reacted and unreacted silver bromide crystals; this latent image is transformed by processing into a permanent visible image.

1.3.5 Processing

The latent image is made visible by chemical processing, the active stages being developing and fixing (Box 1.9). These can be controlled manually, or

Fig. 1.9 Panoramic extra-oral cassette containing two intensifying screens and the matching film.

by one of the many processing machines where the transfer of the film through the various stages is automated; the rinse stage is recommended with manual processing.

Box 1.9

Stages of processing an X-ray film
Develop → (Rinse) → Fix → Wash→ Dry

Developing causes the latent image to become visible by converting the exposed silver bromide crystals into silver deposits. Fixing stops this process and removes any unexposed silver bromide crystals, which would otherwise degrade the image, and produces a permanent image displaying the results of the X-ray interactions.

The quality of the final image is strongly dependent on good working practice; the establishment of a quality assurance programme to ensure that high standards are maintained is strongly recommended.

1.3.6   Mounting and storage systems

Radiographs that are not kept and not identifiable as belonging to a particular individual are of no value and cannot aid in the diagnosis and treatment of the patient of whom they were taken. It is critical, therefore, to have a system for storing radiographs, so that they are retrievable and easily identifiable.

There are a number of commercially available accessories for both mounting and storing dental radiographs. Mounting systems range from simple acetate sheets to purpose-designed mounts for specific arrangements of films, often surrounded by black-out material. Storage systems generally utilize envelopes which may be designed to be an integral part of the patient's record or filed separately; various commercial systems are available to help with this. All the available systems have their advocates, and it is a matter of personal preference which is utilized. The key to each must be that there is sufficient information to identify to whom the radiographs refer and when they were taken.

Radiographic images need to be kept for a substantial period of time, in order to comply with national and European directives. The Consumer Protection Act[3] indicates that records should be retained until 27 years of age, or 11 years after the last record entry.

1.3.7   Viewing systems

Radiographic images should be viewed using transmitted light, through the radiograph, preferably from a viewing box (Chapter 4, Fig. 4.1). This enables the different levels of greyness to be fully appreciated and the contrast between adjacent structures to be clearly seen. The usual system is to have a bright white light illuminating an opalescent screen upon which the radiograph can be placed for viewing. More detailed consideration of the influence of the viewing conditions is dealt with in Chapter 3 (Fig. 3.6).

1.   The Ionising Radiations Regulations 1985, and Approved Code of Practice; The Ionising Radiation (Protection of Persons Undergoing Medical Examination or Treatment) Regulations, 1988.

2. *Guidelines on Radiology Standards for Primary Dental Care* (1994). Documents of the NRPB, Vol. 5, No. 3.

3. Consumer Protection Act (1987). London, HMSO.

2 Radiographic projections and anatomical features

2.1	INTRODUCTION	18
2.2	RADIOGRAPHIC PROJECTIONS	18
	2.2.1 Intra-oral views	**19**
	2.2.2 Extra-oral views	**22**
2.3	LISTS OF ANATOMICAL FEATURES	31
	2.3.1 Coding	**32**
	2.3.2 Explanatory notes	**38**

2 Radiographic projections and anatomical features

2.1 INTRODUCTION

A knowledge of the normal anatomy of a region and its radiological appearance is essential as a basis for radiological examination, in order to aid the recognition of abnormal features. A good working knowledge can also enable the examiner to *fast forward* to the final stage of considering the detailed examination of any suspected abnormalities.

This chapter concentrates on normal anatomical features and their appearance in those radiographic views that are most widely used in dentistry. Each of the views used has a section in which the clinical indications and a number of important technical points are summarized. The descriptive sections on teeth, the mandible, maxilla, other hard tissue structures, soft tissue structures, and air spaces highlight key points about the anatomy, as it influences the radiological image. All features illustrated in this chapter are listed in these anatomical groupings, which matches the manner in which anatomical knowledge is frequently recalled. Each feature mentioned is coded with an alphanumeric notation, which is reproduced in Appendix B.

2.2 RADIOGRAPHIC PROJECTIONS

The following views are included in this chapter:

Intra-oral:
- Bitewings
- Periapicals
- Occlusals
  — oblique
  — cross-sectional

Extra-oral:
- Panoramic
- Oblique lateral and bimolar
- Lateral cephalometric
- Other extra-oral views
  — occipitomental (OM)
  — postero-anterior mandible (PA mandible)
  — submentovertex (submentovertical, SMV)

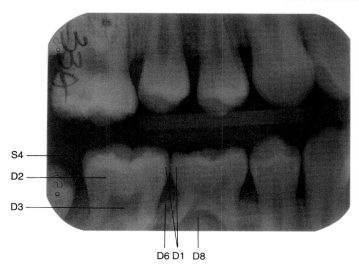

S4

D2

D3

D6 D1 D8

Fig. 2.1 R bitewing radiograph of mixed dentition: F 10.

2.2.1 Intra-oral views

Bitewings

Clinical indications

1. Detection of carious lesions, primary and secondary.
2. Determination of depth of carious lesions.
3. Demonstration of alveolar bone level in cases of mild to moderate chronic inflammatory periodontal disease.
4. Demonstration of restorations; excesses and defects.

Technical points

Head position: ala-tragus line parallel to the floor to ensure occlusal plane parallel to floor (or at 90° with supine patient).

Film position: lingual, and parallel, to the teeth being examined, held in position by a tab or a film holder.

Centring point: opposite lower first molar; indicated on outside of face by placing anterior edge of cylindrical or rectangular cone in line with corner of mouth.

Horizontal angle: at 90° to the line of the arch; indicated by the line of the lower jaw or a finger held in line with the teeth. Looking down on the tube from above verifies that open end of cone is parallel to the chosen line.

Vertical angle:
— adult teeth   + 10° ⎫
— deciduous teeth + 5° ⎬ to the occlusal plane
— *or* determined by film holder indicating device.

Periapicals

Clinical indications

1. Detection of periapical or para-radicular bone change.
2. Pre-endodontic and pre-extraction evaluation — number and morphology; proximity to anatomical structures.

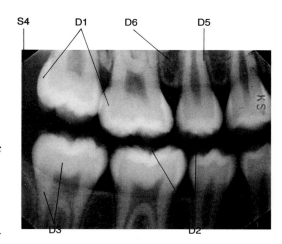

S4   D1   D6   D5

D3   D2

Fig. 2.2 R bitewing radiograph of adult dentition: M 15.

3. Determination of alveolar bone support.
4. Localization of unerupted teeth, pathological lesions, or foreign objects.
5. Post-trauma.
6. Review of clinical/surgical procedures.

Technical points

Two techniques are available for taking periapical radiographs:

(1) paralleling
(2) bisecting angle

In both periapical techniques the raised dot on the film packet should be placed towards the occlusal plane, except when examining lower right third molars when it should be placed towards the front of the mouth; in this position it is least likely to obscure a critical part of the image.

Paralleling

Film position: film packet positioned parallel to the long axis of the tooth, and to the segment of the arch. This requires a film holder of which a variety are available, all of which incorporate a bite block and film support, and an indicator arm which assists in aligning the tube. Some have, in addition, a locator ring attached to the indicator arm. The most important point when taking paralleling periapicals is to position the film packet correctly; it will normally be some distance from the tooth; cotton wool rolls can assist with stabilization of the film holder but must be placed between the bite block and the opposing teeth, otherwise the portion of film available to record an image is reduced.

Centring point, horizontal, and vertical angles: all determined by the film holder.

Bisecting angle

Head position:
— upper teeth: ala-tragus line parallel to floor (or at 90° with supine patient)
— lower teeth: corner of mouth-tragus line parallel to floor (or at 90° with supine patient), i.e. the head must be tilted further back so as to position the occlusal plane in the correct reference position when the mouth is slightly open.

Film position: film packet is held against the crown of the tooth being examined, naturally making an angle with the tooth's long axis, as a result of the intervening hard and soft tissues that surround the root. The film packet can be supported by film holders or the patient.

Centring points: opposite the required apex on the following lines:
— upper teeth: on the ala-tragus line
— lower teeth: 1 cm above the lower border of the mandible

Horizontal angle: at 90° to the tangent to the relevant arch segment.

Vertical angle: the angle formed by the long axis of the tooth and the plane of the film packet is mentally bisected; the central ray is directed at 90° to this bisector; positive for upper teeth, negative for lower (i.e. directed towards the occlusal plane). For lower third molars a small positive angle (+5°) is often appropriate, due to the lingual inclination of the second and third molars (curve of Monson).

Occlusals

There are two categories of occlusal radiographs:

(1)   oblique
(2)   cross-sectional

The difference is in the relationship of the central X-ray beam to the long axis of the teeth being examined. In both categories the film packet is placed in the occlusal plane, with the raised dot at the front of the mouth, away from any region of interest.

Oblique

Oblique occlusal radiographs utilize the bisecting angle principle, as in the bisecting angle periapical technique; the central ray is therefore at an oblique angle to the long axes of the teeth. The term 'topographical occlusal' refers to oblique occlusals. The image of the teeth is equivalent to the periapical image, covering a larger area.

Clinical indications

1.   Determination of presence or absence of developing teeth, and supernumeraries.
2.   Situations where periapicals are desirable but cannot be obtained (e.g. where mouth opening is limited).
3.   Situations where periapical pathology is present, and of such a size that it is not demonstrated on a single periapical view (e.g. cystic lesions).
4.   In situations where it is advantageous for the patient to support the film packet in the occlusal plane (e.g. young children, handicapped patients, trauma cases, and patients unable to tolerate conventionally placed periapical film packets).

Technical points

Head position: same as for bisecting angle periapicals.

Centring points: due to the larger film area to be covered compared with periapicals, these are further from the occlusal plane:
—   upper teeth: 1 cm above the ala-tragus line
—   lower teeth: through lower border of mandible

Horizontal angle: at 90° to a tangent to the relevant arch segment except where this would mean the central ray passing through the zygoma, when the beam must be angled to avoid this dense bone.

Vertical angle: determined according to the bisecting angle principle. The film is always in the occlusal plane so angles will be greater than for equivalent periapicals.

Cross-sectional

Cross-sectional occlusal radiographs are those where the central X-ray beam is directed along the long axes of the teeth. In the mandible this is relatively straightforward and there are many applications. In the maxilla the technique, known as the vertex occlusal, requires the x-ray beam to pass through the cranium and the eyes; for this reason it should not be the technique of choice, and must only be taken using a special cassette fitted with intensifying screens, and matching screen film. The term '*true* occlusal' is also appropriate for lower cross-sectional occlusals as the central ray is directed at 90°, or *true*, to the film.

Clinical indications

Mandible:
1. Bucco-lingual localization of unerupted teeth, pathology, and foreign objects.
2. Demonstration of bucco-lingual expansion caused by pathological change.
3. Demonstration of radiopaque calculi in submandibular gland salivary ducts.

Maxilla, only if other views are not considered appropriate:
1. Comparison of the right and left side of the hard palate in cases of pathological change.
2. Bucco-palatal relationship of unerupted teeth, pathological lesions, and foreign objects.

Technical points

Mandible:
Head position: the head must be tilted further back in order to allow room for the X-ray tube head at the required position.

Centring points: centre over the area of interest; this will often be an erupted reference tooth.

Angulation: the central ray is directed at 90° to the film (the occlusal plane)

Maxilla: To take a vertex occlusal radiograph (Fig. 2.13) a special cassette *must* be used, with a matching screen-film combination. This technique will not be described as its use is limited, and not generally appropriate for dental practice.

Intra-oral radiographs provide particularly clear images of the anatomical features included in the field of view. Figures 2.1–2.22 show a selection of bitewing, periapical, and occlusal views, with a number of anatomical features identified by their codes; individual teeth are referred to using the FDI notation, which is used throughout the text (see Chapter 3, p. 55 for explanation).

2.2.2   Extra-oral views

The extra-oral views illustrating this chapter are detailed below: clinical indications for their use are noted; technical points are not provided except where they assist in understanding and interpreting the image. Appropriate sized cassettes with fast screen–film combinations must be used for all extra-oral radiography, together with specialized X-ray equipment.

Panoramic

The panoramic radiograph provides an image of the dental arches, and structures immediately above and below them, incorporating only those structures within an 'image layer'; the layer is designed to incorporate the dental arches, and features in close proximity to the teeth; structures remote from the teeth will not produce clear, recognizable images, unless they are very dense structures. The technique is complex and operator positioning of the patient critical

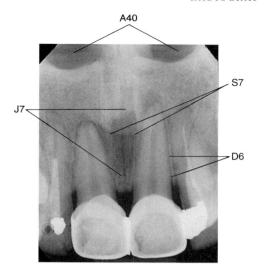

Fig. 2.3   Bisecting angle periapical centred on 11/21; 12 and 22 have been root treated; periapical areas of inflammatory bone resorption related to 21 and 22. The line caused by the tip of the nose is particularly clear and crosses teeth and interdental bone: M 44.

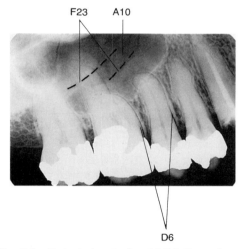

Fig. 2.5   Periapical centred on 16/15; the outline of the maxillary sinus is clear except where it crosses roots of teeth; within the image of the sinus are narrow, parallel radiolucent lines caused by neurovascular channels within the wall of the sinus.

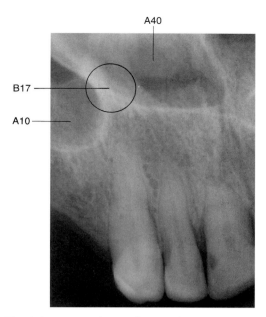

Fig. 2.4   Periapical centred on 13; the junction of the outlines of the nasal cavity and the maxillary sinus is referred to as the Y-line of Ennis. First described by Ennis who recognized the characteristic shape as similar to an upside down Y, it is sometimes portrayed as an X.

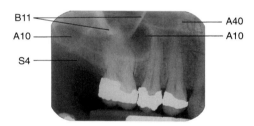

Fig. 2.6   Periapical centred on 16: M 10.

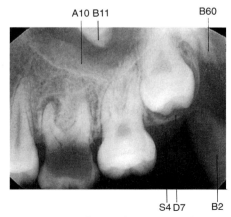

Fig. 2.7   Periapical centred on 27; note the presence and position of the coronoid process: F 24.

for good quality images. The X-ray beam passes through the jaws from lingual to buccal, and is directed at a slight upward angulation with respect to the occlusal plane, for the same reason that the beam is directed downwards in bitewing radiography.

Clinical indications

Demonstration of the complete dentition and supporting structures for:

1. Determination of presence, absence, location, etc., of the dental structures.

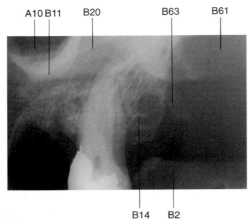

A10 B11   B20   B63   B61

B14   B2

Fig. 2.8   Periapical centred on 28; the pterygoid plates and hamulus are seen when the film is positioned well back in the mouth; the coronoid process is at the foot of the image with the mouth wide open.

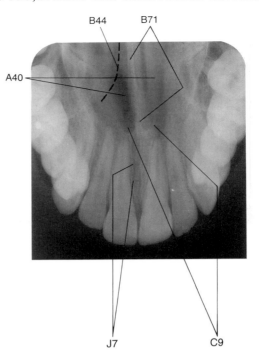

B44   B71

A40

J7   C9

Fig. 2.9   Upper anterior oblique occlusal: M 14.

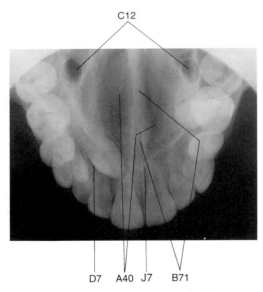

C12

D7 A40 J7 B71

Fig. 2.10   Upper anterior oblique occlusal; a steeper vertical angle brings upper opening of naso-lacrimal ducts into field of view: F 14.

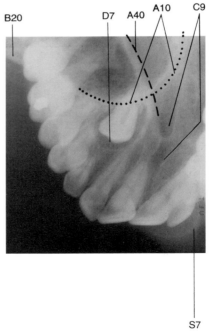

B20   D7   A40   A10   C9

S7

Fig. 2.11   Upper oblique occlusal centred on 13: M 14.

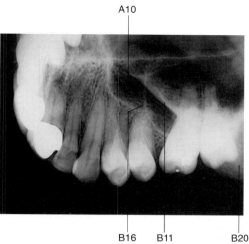

Fig. 2.12 Upper oblique occlusal centred on 25: F 25.

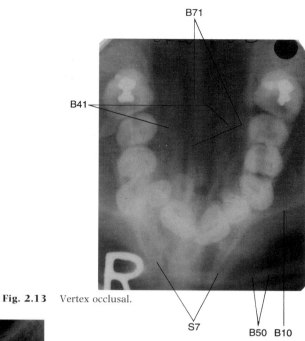

Fig. 2.13 Vertex occlusal.

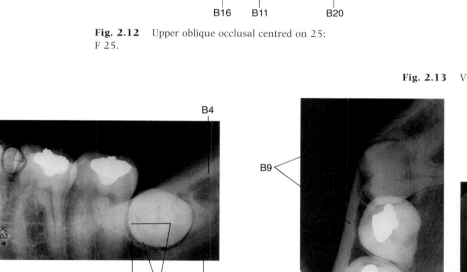

Fig. 2.14 Periapical and cross-sectional occlusal, using a periapical film packet, of transverse 38: M 29.

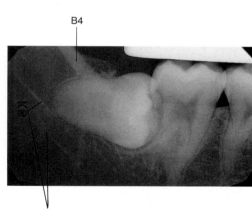

Fig. 2.15 Periapical of 48: M 22.

2. Determination of pathology within the bone and the extent of such pathology.

3. Demonstration of the height of the supporting alveolar bone.

4. Demonstration of fractures, their presence and displacement.

5. Review following surgery or treatment of fracture cases.

When examining the panoramic image it can be considered as having three main segments. The anterior region from canine to canine is seen as if looking straight on at the patient; each molar region and ramus is seen as if looking from the side of the patient. The premolar regions are at the crossover between the two. Understanding the changing nature of this projection is useful when anticipating and recognizing the anatomical features.

The sequence of images in Fig. 2.23 shows a panoramic radiograph of a 17-year-old female, with supporting outline tracings of the features that can be

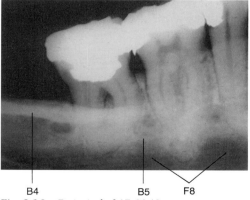

Fig. 2.16 Periapical of 47: M 40.

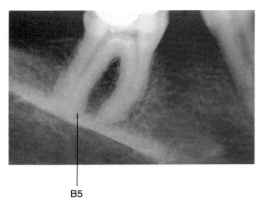

B5

Fig. 2.17   Periapical of 47: M 41.

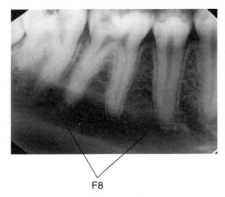

F8

Fig. 2.18   Periapical of 46: F 17.

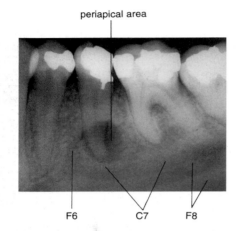

periapical area

F6   C7   F8

Fig. 2.19   Periapical of 35: F 32.

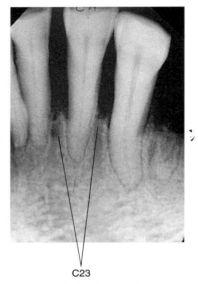

C23

Fig. 2.20   Periapical of lower incisors, with horizontal bone loss due to periodontal disease: F 75.

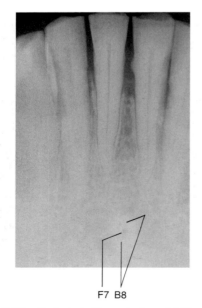

F7 B8

Fig. 2.21   Periapical of lower incisors: M 49.

accurately identified; the alphanumeric codes are superimposed on the anatomical features represented. The clarity of individual features is variable from patient to patient, in particular with respect to the inferior dental (ID) canal and mental foramen, and in response to muscle attachments: a selection of variations is shown in Fig. 2.24.

Oblique lateral and bimolar views

The oblique lateral view provides an image of a section of one side of the jaws, and is predominantly used to examine the mandible. It can be taken using a dental x-ray machine in conjunction with an extra-oral cassette. The patient's head is rotated to place the arch section to be examined parallel to the film; the further the head is rotated the more anterior the field of view. The bimolar is a variation of the technique to show the upper and lower teeth equally, and can be used in small children as an alternative to bitewing radiographs.

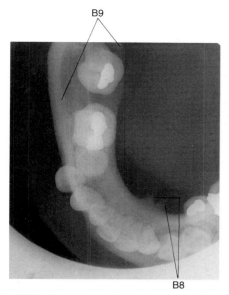

Fig. 2.22 Cross-sectional occlusal of right side of mandible: F 33.

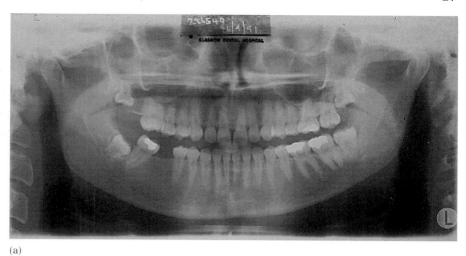

(a)

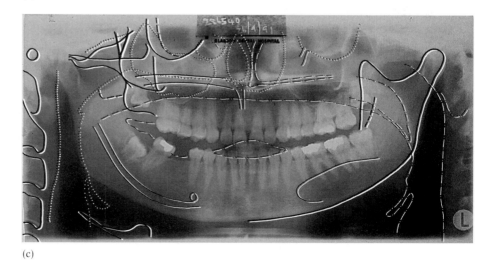

(c)

Fig. 2.23
(a) Panoramic radiograph: F 17.
(b) Alphanumeric codes superimposed on anatomical features.
(c) Outline tracing of features.

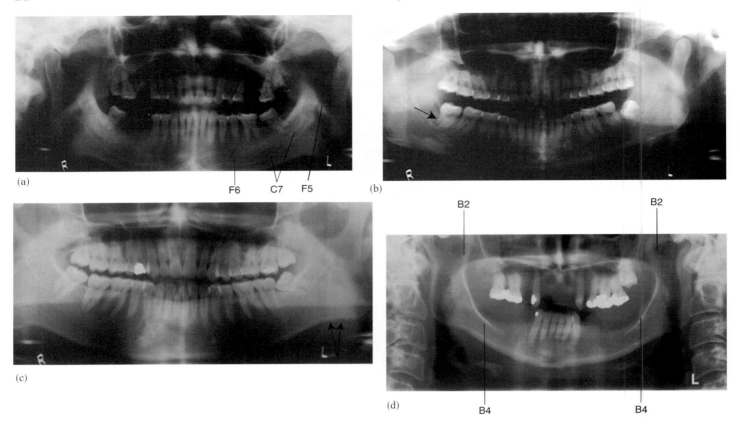

Fig. 2.24
(a) Clear inferior dental (ID) canal and mental foramen: F 36. (b) Unusual appearance of subsidiary canal branching off to 48: F 20. (c) Ridged lower border related to attachment of masseter muscle (arrowed): M 21. (d) Prominent external oblique ridges and coronoid processes: F 47.

Clinical indications

The clinical indications for a panoramic radiograph are also valid for the oblique lateral view. In addition, this view is particularly useful in the following situations:

1. Where a panoramic radiograph is not available, not possible, or impractical.

2. When it is important to incorporate the full bucco-lingual depth of the mandible when imaging an extensive pathological lesion.

3. When the improved detail provided by a static image, is required.

Figure 2.25 illustrates the use of this view in examining an impacted third molar.

Lateral cephalometric

The lateral cephalometric radiograph (Fig. 2.26) is a true lateral view of the facial bones, base of skull, and upper cervical spine, of particular value in analyzing jaw relationships. The radiograph is taken in a standardized manner with regard to the head position, and its relation to the X-ray source and central ray; this enables comparison with precisely similar projections to be made of the same, and different persons. Current good radiation hygiene practice recommends that the X-ray beam be collimated so as to avoid unnecess-

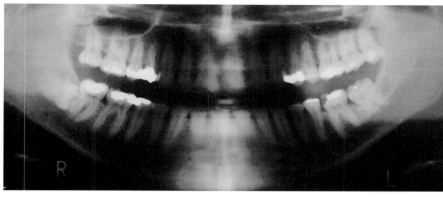

(a)

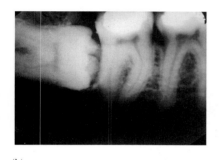

(b)

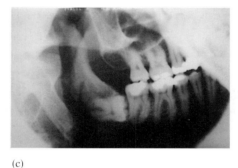

(c)

Fig. 2.25
(a) Panoramic radiograph fails to clearly demonstrate precise morphological details of 48 root mass: M 32.
(b) Periapical film is not far enough back in the mouth to show the apices.
(c) The oblique lateral view provides a clear image of the shape of the two roots, and their relationship with the ID canal.

arily exposing parts of the head that are not required for the subsequent analysis.* The full name is often abbreviated to lateral ceph., and this form will be used in text captions. The clinical indications for its use are related to appearance as well as function, and it is important to visualize the soft tissue profile in the same image as the underlying hard tissue structures; this is achieved by placement of an aluminium filter between the source and the patient to reduce the intensity of the beam before it passes through the soft tissues.

Clinical indications

1. Orthodontic patients, particularly those with a probable skeletal discrepancy between the dental bases, or requiring fixed appliance therapy.

2. Pre-treatment planning, and post-surgery review for orthognathic surgery patients.

3. Implant planning.

Other extra-oral views

In general dental, and specialist orthodontic, practice the various views referred to in the first part of this chapter, and illustrated in Figs 2.1–2.26, are those that are likely to be routinely available. There are a number of other views, however, that may be taken in hospital situations as part of the investigation of disorders outside the strictly dental sphere. The following selection of views has been included, so that the practitioner with access to them, even infrequently, has a reference image to aid in their examination:

* Report of a Joint Working Party of the British Society for the Study of Orthodontics and the British Society of Dental and Maxillofacial Radiology (1985). The reduction of the dose to patients during lateral cephalometric radiology. *British Journal of Orthodontics*, **12**, 176–8.

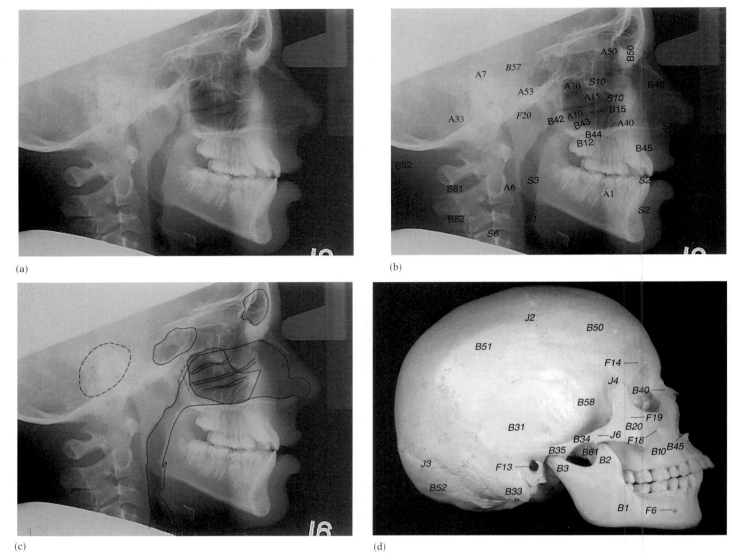

Fig. 2.26
(a) Lateral ceph.: M 12.
(b) Alphanumeric codes superimposed on anatomical features.
(c) Outline tracing of features.
(d) Equivalent photographic view of a skull.

1.   Occipitomental (OM)

2.   Postero-anterior mandible (PA mandible)

3.   Submentovertex (submentovertical, SMV)

Occipitomental (OM)
This radiographic projection is taken to demonstrate the middle third of the face, including the maxillary sinus, orbit, frontal sinus, and zygomatic complex of both sides. It is a postero-anterior (PA) projection; the beam passes through the patient from the posterior aspect to the anterior aspect, in order to place the features of interest as close to the film as possible, thus minimizing the magnification that is caused by the divergent nature of the X-ray beam.

Clinical indications in the field of dentistry

1.   Suspected maxillary sinus pathology.

2.   Mid-facial pain of unknown cause.

3.   Trauma to the middle third of the face.

Figure 2.27 is an occipitomental view of an adult patient suffering from left facial discomfort of indeterminate cause. Important anatomical features have been identified.

Postero-anterior mandible (PA mandible)
This projection is the equivalent for the mandible of the occipitomental view for the middle third of the face. It can be taken using a cephalostat (PA ceph.), or a conventional skull unit.

Clinical indications in the field of dentistry

1.   Ectopic teeth in the posterior body and ramus of the mandible.

2.   Determination of the extent, and involvement of other structures, of pathology in the mandible.

3.   Trauma to the lower part of the face.

4.   Evaluation of asymmetry.

Figure 2.28 is a PA view of the complete head of a teenager with multiple cystic lesions in the jaws (the case is discussed further in Chapter 8, Fig. 8.15). In situations where the expected abnormality is likely to be confined to the mandible, the X-ray beam will be collimated to prevent exposure of the vault of the skull.

Submentovertex (submentovertical, SMV)
This projection provides a view of the head as if looking from underneath. This view can be used to demonstrate the base of the skull, the plan profile of the mandible, and the zygomatic arches, for which reduced exposure factors are needed to prevent over-penetration.

Clinical indications

1.   Pre-treatment planning for orthognathic surgery patients.

2.   Determination of bucco-lingual position of impacted lower third molars, displaced in the ramus.

3.   Demonstration of bucco-lingual expansion or destruction, by pathological lesions.

4.   Investigation of obscure pain indicative of a disorder of the mandibular division of the trigeminal nerve (to demonstrate foramen ovale).

5.   Trauma to the zygomatic arches. In this situation, this projection must only be taken if it has been verified radiologically that there is no cervical spine damage.

Figure 2.29 illustrates an SMV radiograph of a young adult with mandibular asymmetry; the shape of the mandible is clearly seen from the buccal and lingual cortical outlines. The zygomatic arches are not seen as the exposure is adequate in this case to show the basal foramina.

2.3   LISTS OF ANATOMICAL FEATURES

The lists following are reproduced in Appendix B. The alphanumeric coding is used to identify the features marked on the radiographs illustrating this chapter, and will be found on illustrations elsewhere in the book when an anatomical feature is being highlighted. The radiological visualization of any

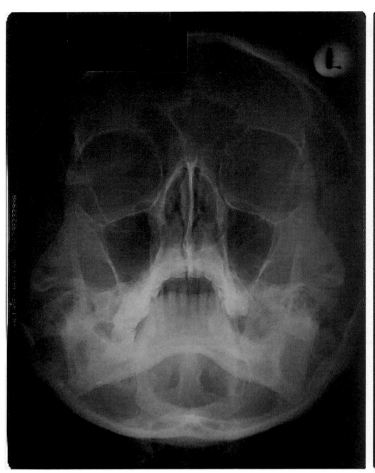

(a)

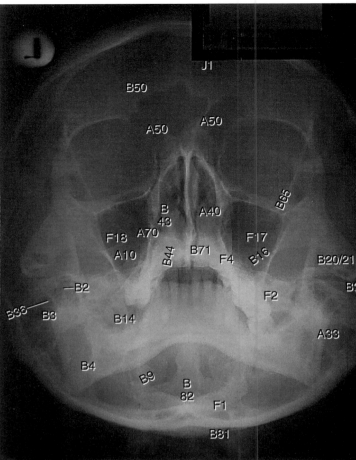

(b)

anatomical feature is dependent on its presence, the quality of the X-ray beam, and the geometrical relationship with the X-ray beam. Fine features, such as sutures, are often not well depicted, although they are easily found when examining a dry skull; these features are, however, incorporated in the following lists as they can then be used to assist in examining skeletal material as well as radiographs.

2.3.1   Coding

D   =   dental structures
B   =   bones and bony features
J   =   joints, including sutures
A   =   air spaces
F   =   fissures, foramina, and depressions
C   =   canals
S   =   soft tissues

Some features fall into more than one grouping; they are listed in both groups but have one code, derived from the most appropriate group.

Dental structures

D1   Enamel
D2   Dentine

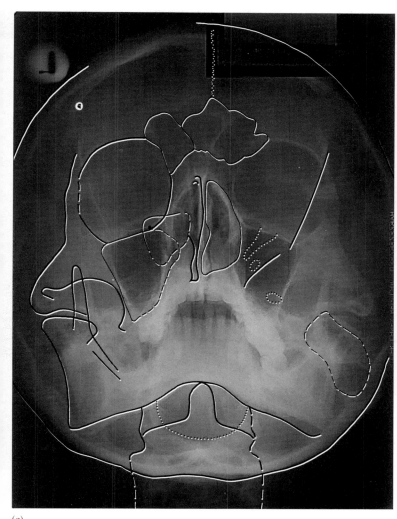

(c)

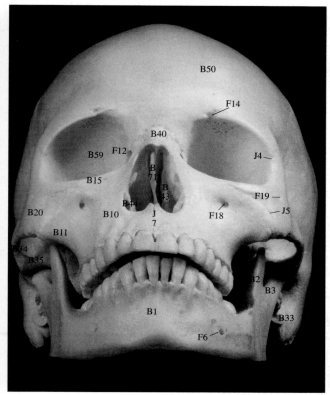

(d)

Fig. 2.27
(a) OM view: F 33.
(b) Alphanumeric codes superimposed on anatomical features.
(c) Outline tracing of features.
(d) Equivalent photographic view of a skull.

D3	Pulp chamber	
D4	Cementum	
D5	Periodontal ligament space	
D6	Lamina dura of tooth socket	
D7	Follicle (follicular space)	
D8	Tooth germ	
D9	Tooth crypt	

Bones and bony features

B1	Mandible :	coronoid process	B2
		condylar process	B3
		external oblique ridge	B4
		mylohyoid ridge	B5
		lingula	B6
		ID canal	C7
		mental protuberance	B7
		genial tubercles	B8
		cortical margin	B9
B10	Maxilla:	zygomatic process	B11
		hard palate	B12
		— ghost image	B13

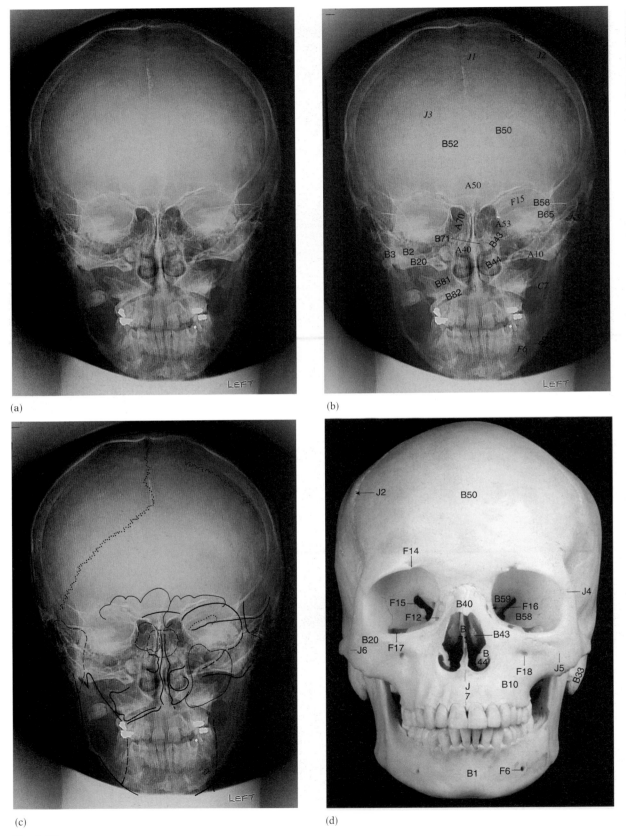

Fig. 2.28
(a) PA view of the head: F 16. (b) Alphanumeric codes superimposed on anatomical features. (c) Outline tracing of features. (d) Equivalent photographic view of a skull.

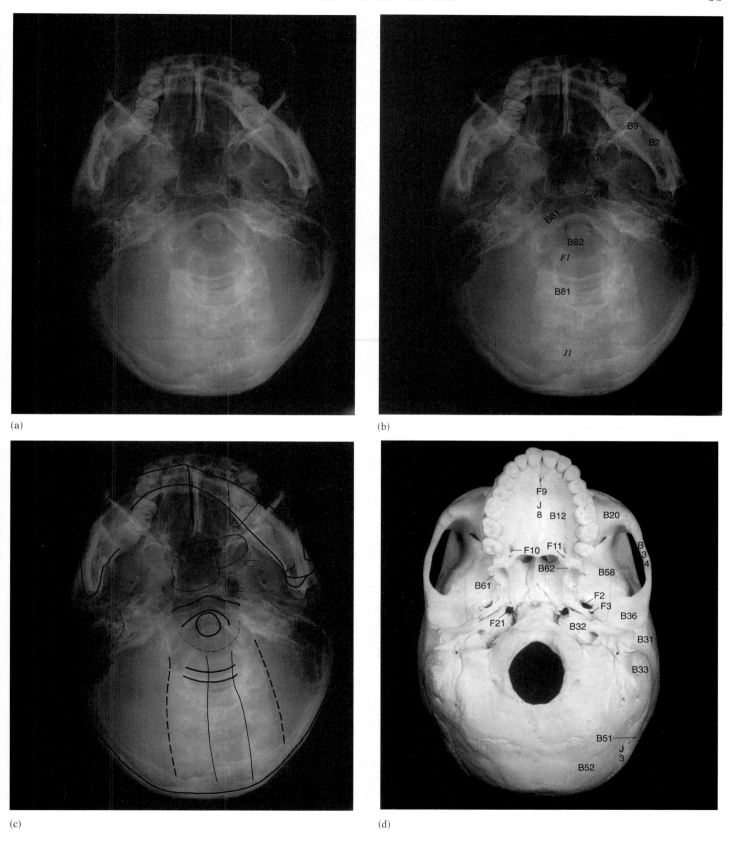

Fig. 2.29
(a) SMV view: F 24. (b) Alphanumeric codes superimposed on anatomical features. (c) Outline tracing of features. (d) Equivalent photographic view of a skull.

		tuberosity	B14
		inferior margin orbit	B15
		antral septum	B16
		Y-line of Ennis	B17
		canine fossa	B18
B20	Zygoma:	temporal process	B21
B26	Hyoid bone		
B30	Temporal:	squamous	B31
		petrous	B32
		mastoid process	B33
		zygomatic process	B34
		— articular eminence	B35
		glenoid fossa	B36
		styloid process	B37
B40	Nasal:	turbinate bones	B41
		— superior	B42
		— middle	B43
		— inferior	B44
		anterior nasal spine	B45
		nasal septum (vomer)	B71
B50	Frontal		
B51	Parietal		
B52	Occipital		
B53	Sphenoid:	clinoid processes	B54
		— anterior	B55
		— posterior	B56
		sella turcica	B57
		greater wing	B58
		lesser wing	B59
		pterygoid plates	B60
		— lateral	B61
		— medial	B62
		— hamulus	B63
		spine	B64
		innominate line	B65
B70	Ethmoid:	vomer (nasal septum)	B71
		crista galli	B72
B80	cervical spine:	C1 (atlas)	B81
		C2 (axis)	B82

Joints, including sutures

J1	Sagittal suture
J2	Coronal suture
J3	Lambdoid suture

Various sutures between facial bones:

J4	zygomatico-frontal
J5	zygomatico-maxillary
J6	zygomatico-temporal
J7	median maxillary
J8	median palatine
D5	periodontal ligament
J9	temporo-mandibular joint
J10	mandibular symphysis (until fused)

Air spaces

A10	Maxillary sinus
A33	Mastoid air cells
A40	Nasal cavity
A50	Frontal sinus
A53	Sphenoid sinus
A70	Ethmoid air cells
A80	Pharynx

Fissures, foramina, and depressions

F1	F. magnum
F2	F. ovale
F3	F. spinosum
F4	F. rotundum
F5	Mandibular foramen
F6	Mental foramen
F7	Lingual foramen
F8	Submandibular fossa
F9	Incisive foramen
F10	Greater palatine foramen
F11	Lesser palatine foramen
F12	Superior opening of lacrimal duct
F13	External auditory meatus
F14	Supra-orbital foramen
F15	Superior orbital fissure
F16	Optic foramen
F17	Inferior orbital fissure
F18	Infra-orbital foramen
F19	Zygomatic foramen
F20	Pterygo-maxillary fissure
F21	F. lacerum
F22	Grooves for meningeal vessels
F23	Grooves/canals for nutrient vessels, and miscellaneous neurovascular bundles

Canals

C7	Inferior dental (alveolar) canal
C9	Nasopalatine canal
C12	Lacrimal duct
C23	Nutrient canals

Soft tissues

S1	Tongue
S2	Lips
S3	Soft palate
S4	Gingiva
S5	Epiglottis
S6	Posterior pharyngeal wall
S7	Nose
S8	Ear lobes
S9	Eyes
S10	Eyelids

2.3.2   Explanatory notes

- Dental structures
- Bones and bony features
  - mandible
  - maxilla
  - other hard tissue structures
- Joints, including sutures
- Air spaces
- Fissures, foramina, and depressions
- Canals
- Soft tissues

Dental structures

The teeth comprise the hard tissues enamel, dentine, and cementum, and the connective tissue components of the pulp within the pulp chamber. Dentine and cementum have a different microscopic structure, but the same effective atomic number and are indistinguishable on radiographs. It is only when there is an excess of cementum on the outer surface of the root that it is recognizable due to the resultant altered root shape. Enamel has a higher atomic number than dentine and cementum, due to its greater degree of mineralization and is more radiopaque. The contents of the pulp chamber have little effect on the X-ray beam and an empty pulp chamber looks essentially the same as one containing a vital pulp; it is mainly for this reason that it is more correct to refer to the 'pulp chamber' rather than the 'pulp' when discussing the radiographic image.

Teeth are normally only present when attached to bone; the supporting tissues therefore fall naturally within this section. The periodontal ligament fibres connect cementum to the thin cortical bone of the socket prior to and after eruption; superficially, they attach to the gingiva around the neck of the erupted tooth. The fibres themselves do not show up in radiographic images. In common with the philosophy applied to the pulp chamber it is therefore correct to refer to the 'periodontal ligament space'.

All unerupted teeth in which crown formation is complete have a soft tissue covering to their crown, commonly known as the follicle. This represents the reduced enamel epithelium and on eruption it blends with the oral epithelium and then disappears. It is the bony crypt containing the follicle that is actually seen, and the 'follicular space' between the crypt and the enamel.

Bones and bony features

Mandible

The mandible is a single bone which develops in two halves, the right and left sides uniting at about one year of age; prior to that time non-mineralized connective tissue is present between the two halves at the mandibular symphysis, and is seen as a linear radiolucency. The mandible consists of basal bone and alveolar bone, the latter providing support for the teeth. The basal bone can be divided into two main regions, the body and the ramus, with the angle of the mandible forming their junction. The ramus has two processes, the condylar process, which contributes to the temporo-mandibular joint, and the coronoid process, which provides attachment for the temporalis muscle. The bone is of two types; cancellous bone with a cortical covering of variable thickness according to the section of the jaw. Cancellous bone consists of bone trabeculae and intervening soft tissues; the trabeculae attenuate the X-ray beam to a considerable extent, appearing white or radiopaque. The intervening non-mineralized connective tissues, and bone marrow, appear relatively radiolucent. This combination of hard and soft tissues results in a pattern which is seen throughout the mandible and is subject to considerable variation as a result of factors such as age, stress, and related pathology. The cortical bony covering is of variable thickness according to the particular site; in general the thickness is greatest in the body region of the mandible, and is normally symmetrical.

A number of muscles originate from or insert into the mandible, including the major muscles of mastication; the temporalis, masseter, and medial and lateral pterygoids. Smooth bone provides relatively little purchase for muscle attachments. The necessary holding power is obtained by areas of increased roughness or ridges of bone. Features such as this may be evident as areas of increased opacity, due to for example:

Increased roughness: the angle region of the mandible where masseter and medial pterygoid both insert.

Ridges of bone: the external oblique ridge where the tendon and lower fibres of temporalis insert.

Maxilla

There are two maxillae, a right and a left, which constitute the upper jaw, forming a large part of the middle third of the face. Like the mandible, each maxilla has two major functional components, the dento-alveolar portion and the basal portion, containing the maxillary air sinus, or antrum (also known as the antrum of Highmore). In addition because of the complex bony architecture of the face there are numerous processes which reach out to other bones in order to unite with them at sutures. The two largest processes are the palatine process, the right and left together forming the major part of the hard palate, and the zygomatic process forming the buttress supporting the zygoma (cheek bone).

The bone of the maxilla is predominantly cancellous with a much thinner covering of cortical bone than is seen in the mandible. There are no canals directly equivalent to the inferior dental canal. The major neurovascular bundles run along the walls of the sinuses where they often cause parallel-sided radiolucent images, without cortical margins; the intra-bony course is directly through cancellous bone.

The sinuses contain air and as such are radiolucent unless the path of the X-ray beam is through a greater than normal thickness of other tissues, or the sinus contents are altered due to inflammation or some other pathological process. Each sinus is a single cavity which opens into the middle meatus of the nasal cavity quite high up on the medial wall of the antrum. The antrum is frequently partially divided by antral septa which normally arise from the floor extending upwards. The septa are thin plates of bone which result in thin radiopaque lines. When incompletely shown on a radiograph, this line adjacent to the radiolucency of the sinus can mimic the appearance of a cystic lesion, which is important when considering the differential diagnosis of antral 'radiolucencies'.

The 'Y-line of Ennis' is the name used to describe the confluence of the radiopaque lines forming the boundaries of the maxillary sinus, and the nasal cavity. The appearance is often of an inverted Y, and was first described by Ennis; a common alternative is an X shape.

Other hard tissue structures

The majority of structures seen on dental radiographs are part of the mandible or maxilla, but there are sufficient features in close proximity, which belong to other bones to warrant inclusion. These structures are listed according to the bone of origin.

Joints, including sutures

Bones are connected to each other by joints, the majority in the cranio-facial skeleton being sutures. The soft tissue components of joints are not demonstrated by conventional radiographic images, but delineated by the hard tissue boundaries. Special imaging techniques are available to enhance the visibility of the components of the temporo-mandibular joint; these are mentioned in Appendix D.

Air spaces

Air spaces are outlined by virtue of their boundary with adjacent hard or soft tissue. The main air spaces in the vicinity of the teeth and jaws are the oral cavity, the paranasal sinuses, and the pharynx. Air has little effect on the X-ray beam, and is naturally radiolucent. Other structures in the path of the X-ray beam, whether normal or abnormal, soft tissue or hard tissue, will cause some degree of attenuation, and result in varying shades of grey.

The maxillary sinuses are of particular importance to dentists, and some points have been raised in the earlier section on the maxilla. The walls of these sinuses are very thin. It is important to recall this point when examining radiographs and deciding on the posterior extent of the sinus, particularly as demonstrated by panoramic radiographs. A frequent mistake is to identify the opaque line created by the zygomatic process of the maxilla as the sinus margin. Examination of the panoramic image (Fig. 2.23) reveals that the posterior wall of the sinus is relatively vertical, extending upwards from the posterior aspect of the tuberosity. In the presence of a full complement of permanent teeth, the location of the posterior wall will be distal to the third molar.

Fissures, foramina, and depressions

It has already been noted that an increase in the level of opacity of a bone is frequently related to muscle attachments. In contrast, there are also areas where the cross-section of a bone is reduced; this shows up as a reduction in the level of opacity or sometimes as a frank radiolucency. There is an important area in each jaw where this phenomenon occurs.

The most important area in the mandible is the region of the submandibular fossa, where the lingual side of the mandible is hollowed out in relation to the submandibular salivary gland. In the maxilla, the area of interest is the incisive fossa, immediately anterior to the root of the canine, and closely related to the lateral incisor. The radiolucency caused by these depressions can be so intense as to mimic pathological change, such as inflammatory resorption, or even a cystic lesion.

Canals

Numerous canals running through bone, or channels set into bone surfaces, exist to transmit and protect component parts of the various neurovascular bundles. The most important in this region, from a radiological point of view, is the inferior dental (alveolar) canal (ID canal), transmitting the nerve and blood vessels of the same name. The ID canal runs through the mandible from the mandibular foramen, at the site of the lingula, to the mental foramen; a narrow section continues forward transmitting the incisive branch. The canal is made of cortical bone; due to the influence of thickness on image production only images of the two borders in the plane of the X-ray beam are produced, the surfaces more nearly perpendicular to the beam do not show up.

The two borders that may be demonstrated are:

(1)   upper and lower in panoramic and periapical views; and

(2)   buccal and lingual in cross-sectional (plan) views.

The clarity of the images of these borders is influenced by the total thickness of hard tissue in the path of the beam and the relative proportion that the canal contributes. Frequently, only the lower border is seen in panoramic and periapical films, and occasionally none; the lower is the commonly demonstrated border as it is within the thinner part of the mandible, at a level with the submandibular fossa.

Soft tissue structures

Radiographs predominantly demonstrate hard tissue structures due to their relatively high atomic number. Soft tissues will be clearly demarcated either where an interface exists between soft tissue and air, or where there is a considerable thickness of soft tissue in the path of the beam; this may be normal or abnormal tissue.

The tongue and soft palate are particularly important images in the panoramic radiograph where the tongue can be seen to occupy a surprisingly large area. Reference to the section on the panoramic radiograph explains the type of projection each portion of the image provides; the tongue is in very close proximity to the teeth, and will be seen in each of these portions.

3 Examination of radiographs

3.1	INTRODUCTION	44
3.2	CHECKLIST	45
3.3	DETAILS OF COMPONENTS OF CHECKLIST	46
	Background to examination	**46**
	3.3.1 Patient profile	**46**
	3.3.2 Reason for taking the radiograph	**48**
	3.3.3 Radiographic view	**48**
	3.3.4 Technical acceptability	**48**
	3.3.5 Correct viewing conditions	**49**
	Detailed examination	**49**
	3.3.6 Symmetry	**50**
	3.3.7 Margins	**51**
	3.3.8 Bone consistency	**53**
	3.3.9 Dentition	**54**
	3.3.10 Supporting bone	**57**
	3.3.11 Any other features	**58**
	3.3.12 Summary	**65**
	3.3.13 Proposals to meet patient's requirements, including other investigations	**66**
3.4	APPLICATIONS	67

3 Examination of radiographs

3.1 INTRODUCTION

Radiographs are used to provide information that is not usually available by other means. The observer requires certain skills: perceptual, descriptive ability, knowledge, experience, and some common sense. Each of these is important in recognizing radiological features, ascribing a level of importance to the various findings in a single radiograph, and to interpreting them, in conjunction with other available information.

Perceptual and descriptive ability influence how one looks at radiographic images, and translates the visual messages into suitable language for correlation with other information.

Knowledge and experience are gained intentionally, and also subconsciously. The individual's level of knowledge and their breadth of experience both strongly influence how the perceived images are interpreted.

Common sense plays an important role in much decision making, and is particularly relevant to radiological interpretation. The saying 'common things commonly occur' is frequently repeated, and continues to hold true.

There are two frequently used ways of examining a radiograph. The first approach, knowing the reason for taking the radiograph, is to look immediately for the expected information. The panoramic radiograph (Fig. 3.1) was taken for a patient complaining of soreness around the lower wisdom teeth. It

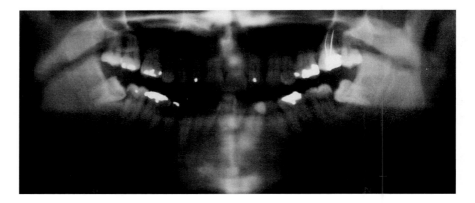

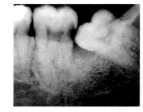

Fig. 3.1 Mesio-angular impacted 38 and 48; caries in distal of 37 and 47 (note short distal roots of 37 and 47 due to resorption): M 25.

is tempting, therefore, to look only for the relevant information in order to decide on an appropriate treatment plan. This radiograph demonstrates the mesio-angular, partially erupted lower third molars, each having two straight roots, their apices situated close to the upper border of the inferior dental (ID) canal. This would be a suitable case for minor oral surgery.

The second approach is to scan the radiograph, looking for something out of the ordinary. Using the same example the caries in the distal surfaces of the lower second molars is quite obvious. Recognition of this situation would influence the patient's treatment plan by postponing the definitive treatment of the third molars until after the second molars have been stabilized.

There is, in addition, a third approach which is to systematically examine all parts of the radiograph. Such a system, which is the one outlined in this chapter, when applied to this same radiograph will ensure that the observer detects the short roots of the lower second molars, and considers possible explanations for this phenomenon, before commencing any treatment plan.

3.2   CHECKLIST

The list below, which is also reproduced as Appendix C, provides one approach to examining radiographs, which the reader should find useful as a basis for development of a personal 'checklist'. Each of the sections presented in this chapter has explanatory notes as to the contribution that it makes to the overall examination of radiographs.

The order suggested for the examination is designed to counteract the instinctive tendency to immediately look at the reason for taking the radiograph, or to concentrate on the most eye-catching area.

A sequential approach is adopted which will ensure coverage of all the information available. The amount of information already known about the patient will vary according to whether they are undergoing regular treatment, or are attending as a casual, or first attender. The apparently long list includes a number of points which can be dealt with routinely, and need not result in an unduly lengthy examination.

Background to examination

1. Patient profile: sex, age, racial or ethnic origin, home environment, diet, dental health care, etc.
2. Reason for taking the radiograph: patient's complaint.
3. Radiographic view: expectation of anatomical features that should be demonstrated.
4. Technical acceptability.
5. Correct viewing conditions:
   — quiet and concentration
   — dim room
   — bright white backlight and masking facilities
   — (magnifying glass)

Detailed examination

6. Symmetry.

7. Margins:
   — continuity
   — width

8. Bone consistency.

9. Dentition:
   — number of teeth
   — eruption status
   — morphology
   — condition

10. Supporting bone:
    — alveolar margins
    — periapical

11. Any other features:
    — radiolucent/radiopaque/combination
    — site
    — shape
    — size
    — margins
    — relation to other structures (?aetiological factors)
    — effect on other structures
    — provisional/differential diagnosis

12. Summary.

13. Proposals to meet patient's requirements, including other investigations.

3.3   DETAILS OF COMPONENTS OF CHECKLIST

Background to examination

3.3.1   Patient profile

Sex, age, racial or ethnic origin, home environment, diet, dental health care, etc. Factors such as these are useful to slot people into definable groups for which normal values or expectations exist. This helps to provide a basis against which variations are readily spotted and opens the way to questioning whether such variations are within normal limits or require further consideration:

Age. The dentition is commonly described as deciduous, mixed, or adult. The age of a patient will indicate to which group they should belong, and will provide a guide to the expected status of the dentition in developmental terms. This presents a backdrop against which 'normal' or 'abnormal' can be ascribed to visually discernible features, for example, an open apex on an upper lateral incisor in an 8-year-old (Fig. 3.2) would be accepted as normal; the same appearance in a 17-year-old (Fig. 3.3) would indicate loss of vitality of the tooth and assist in dating the timing of tooth death. In this example there is evidence in the crown of the tooth of an invagination of the enamel, a condition which predisposes teeth to early loss of vitality resulting from caries developing in the base of the invagination soon after eruption. A similar situation can arise when there is an evagination of pulpal tissue, covered by a thin layer of dentine and enamel which is traumatized by normal function, and easily lost resulting in pulpal exposure (see Chapter 5).

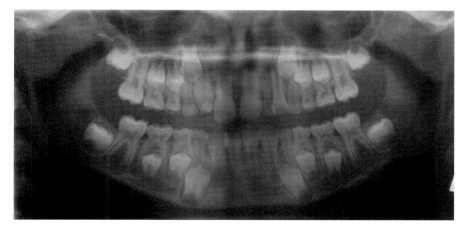

Fig. 3.2 Normal dental development for age; Note the open apices of the erupted incisors and first permanent molars. There is evidence of the third molars developing in each quadrant: the uppers show clear mineralization; 38 has not commenced calcification and 48 has just commenced calcification of two cusps: M 8.

Some diseases have a predilection for particular age groups. The mental prompting needed to consider specific diseases may be initiated by recognition of particular features, for example, irregular but severe alveolar bone loss concentrating on the molars and incisors in a 21-year-old (Fig. 3.4) would suggest a probable diagnosis of juvenile periodontitis.

Sex. Some diseases have a predilection for a particular sex group, whereas others favour neither.

Racial or ethnic origin. An awareness of the influence of ethnic group on the presentation of diseases can assist in ensuring that possible diagnoses are not overlooked. A relevant example of this that is widely accepted is the increased tendency for supernumeraries to be present in some population groups, for example the Chinese as compared to Caucasian Europeans (Fig. 3.5).

Home environment. Dental health is influenced by where people live, their social and educational conditions; location controls external factors such as

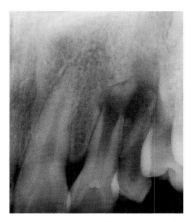

Fig. 3.3 Open apex of 22, associated with invagination: M 17.

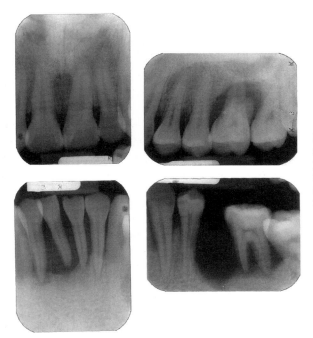

Fig. 3.4 Excessive reduction in height of supporting alveolar bone due to juvenile periodontitis: F 21. The disease is so well established that the effect has spread to involve more teeth than the usual pattern of incisors and first molars: interestingly, the upper incisors have been spared.

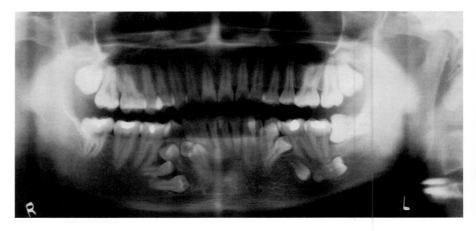

Fig. 3.5 Multiple supernumerary teeth in the premolar region of the mandible: F 20, Chinese.

water fluoridation. People brought up in non-fluoridated areas have a greater chance of suffering from poor dental health as a result of the influence of other factors, than people brought up in regions where the water supply is fluoridated.

Diet. The link between dietary sugar intake and dental caries is proven. Other important influences on the state of the dentition include soft drink intake, and special habits, both voluntary and involuntary, for example, sucking of citrus fruits and bulimia. The oral acid levels resulting from both these examples causes erosion of habitually exposed enamel.

Dental health care. Patients with poor personal dental health care will often have a higher incidence of dental disease. This is an important factor in planning appropriate radiographic investigations, and in particular will influence the timing of review radiographs for regular patients under the ongoing care of a single practitioner.

3.3.2   Reason for taking the radiograph

Knowledge of the clinical reason for requiring the radiographic investigation will provide background information to link with the radiological findings, and will often pose a specific question that needs to be answered. It is important to decide if the question has been adequately answered, and if not plan the next stage of the investigation.

3.3.3   Radiographic view

The most important reason for this is to consider the anatomical features that should be demonstrated, in order to use them as a basis for recognizing variations that may be beyond the range of normal. This particularly applies when examining a radiograph that has been taken by a third person. Chapter 2 deals with the anatomy as depicted on common radiographic views of the teeth and jaws in detail, and a list of anatomical features is provided in Appendix B.

3.3.4   Technical acceptability

The quality of radiographs is influenced by patient factors, radiographic technique factors, and processing factors. Radiographs of poor quality should be retaken, provided the fault is identifiable and can be remedied; there will, however, be occasions where radiographs which are less then perfect still require to be examined, and will still yield useful information. A decision about the quality of the radiograph will help in deciding the level of information that can be retrieved from it.

3.3.5 Correct viewing conditions

(a) *Quiet and concentration.* This facilitates optimum gain from the time available for examining radiographs. Uncontrollable external factors can be distracting, and it is often helpful to arrange the immediate environment in order to optimize concentration; the author utilizes background music to distract from the variable sound level from an adjacent corridor.

(b) *Dim room.* Most people view radiographs in a room that is designed to fulfil other functions, and is often full of a variety of equipment. When the room lights are on it is difficult to prevent visual signals entering the eyes from these other features, which distract from the important object, the radiograph. Concentration is much easier when the main source of visually detectable information is the X-ray viewing box; dimming the room lights wherever possible will assist in this. Where this is quite impractical, such as in the dental surgery during a treatment session, arranging the surgery so that radiographs are examined in a quiet corner, will help to prevent distractions.

(c) *Bright white backlight, and masking facilities.* It is quite possible to detect some of the information in a radiographic image by looking at the film using reflected light, and by holding the film up to the light coming from a window or a light bulb. However, in order to get the maximum possible information it is necessary to use an X-ray viewing box, and have some means of obliterating the light that does not come through the radiograph. Special accessories for this purpose are available. Equally useful, and always available, are patient record cards, or any other opaque object to hand. Another tip that can help is to cup one's hands around the film being examined so that a tunnel is created; a lot of extraneous light is cut out in this way. Figure 3.6 demonstrates the influence that lighting and masking conditions can have; the example used was however considered so poor, as a result of processing faults, that it required a repeat film.

(d) *(Magnifying glass).* Use of a magnifying glass is very much a matter of personal preference. There are situations where enlargement of an image helps the observer to spot something that was previously not evident. There are also many situations where enlargement merely confuses by eliminating the sharpness of an image.

Detailed examination

All of the points covered above influence the quality of information that will be obtained from the radiograph. The explanation of the various factors takes much longer than actually applying the principles that they cover and, once a system has been established, covering these points will become automatic. This can be likened to driving a car. As a learner, individuals consciously acknowledge every action that is needed. Experienced drivers do not need to think consciously, even when carrying out relatively complicated procedures.

In following the system of examination suggested here it is important to develop a strategy, or sequence, that is followed routinely so as not to miss out any aspect of the information to be gained from the radiographic image.

Fig. 3.6a Intra-oral film placed on a viewing box with no masking, normal room lights.

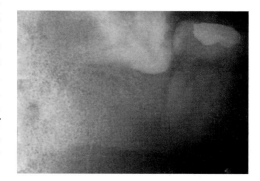

Fig. 3.6b The same film viewed with reflected light.

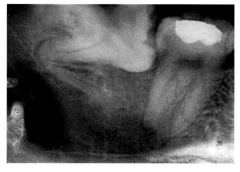

Fig. 3.6c The same film on the viewing box, masked to the area of the film. The sequence of images illustrates how improved visualization of the information present in the emulsion can be gained with proper viewing conditions.

Various systems can be adopted: working from top to bottom, right to left, periphery to centre. Any of these will work, and used in conjunction with the sequence recommended here will increase the interest value of the radiographs, by uncovering unsuspected and often important information.

3.3.6   Symmetry

Compare the same features on the right and left; even when this involves moving from one radiograph to another it is an easy and worthwhile way of spotting differences. If there are no differences then there are most probably no abnormalities, and this will hold true even when examining unfamiliar views provided the patient positioning has been such that the right and left are shown equally. More importantly, if there are differences then the question is raised: 'Are these just normal variations or are they due to abnormalities?' The ability to answer the first part of this question lies in a familiarity with anatomical features, their normal radiological appearance, and the common variations that can occur. If the answer is 'no' or 'I don't know' due to lack of knowledge and/or certainty, then it is important to continue to examine the region in question, and continue on the decision-making pathway.

A number of radiographic views demonstrate both the right and left sides of the patient; three examples which show the right and left sides of the patient in different ways are the panoramic radiograph, bitewing radiographs, and the lateral cephalometric view (Figs 3.7–3.9). The panoramic radiograph shows the two sides separately on a single radiograph in which the geometric factors are the same when imaging the right and the left. The bitewings show equivalent regions on two separate radiographs, as will periapicals of contralateral teeth — there is scope in this situation for the radiographic projection geometry to be different, but when similar the anatomical features can be expected to be essentially symmetrical. In the lateral cephalometric view the right and left sides of the patient are superimposed on each other in the same image; due to the divergence of the X-ray beam the two sides will not match exactly due to the differing amounts of magnification.

One of the fundamental ways of assessing radiographic images of the skeleton is to assess the degree of symmetry between the right and left, the major-

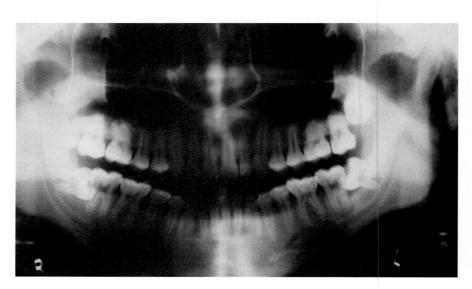

Fig. 3.7   Panoramic radiograph: the dentition is symmetrical except for the angulation of impacted 38 and 48: M 23.

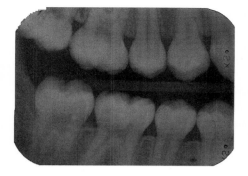 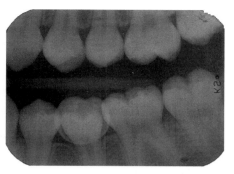

Fig. 3.8   Right and left bitewing radiographs: the obvious asymmetry is in relation to retained 75: F 12.

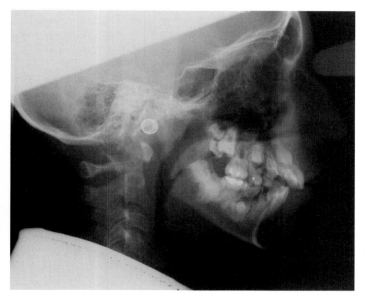

Fig. 3.9   Lateral cephalometric radiograph: F 12. (See also Fig. 3.23.)

ity of body structures being essentially symmetrical. In the region of the facial skeleton the major exception to this is the frontal sinuses which are invariably asymmetrical to some degree (Fig. 3.10). Equivalent projection geometry is necessary for this type of analysis to be carried out with confidence, so the lateral cephalometric view is of limited value.

3.3.7   Margins

(a) Continuity
(b) Width

All structures have margins which are normally continuous. Where they have an identifiable width this may be 'even' or 'progressively changing'; a good example of this is the cortical bony outline of the mandible (see Fig. 3.7). In any view which demonstrates this it will be seen that it normally has an even width within a particular section of the bone, such as the body or ramus; the width in different sections is often dissimilar but should be symmetrical.

Demonstration of the interface between two materials resulting in a clear delineation (clear margins) is influenced by the subject contrast between them, and the relative quantity of each feature in the path of the beam. A good example of a clear delineation is the interface between the tongue and air in

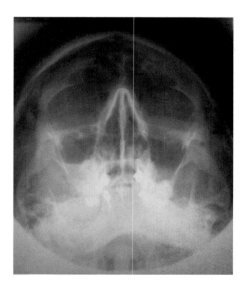

Fig. 3.10   Occipitomental view demonstrating asymmetry of frontal and maxillary sinuses: F 41. The slight asymmetry of the frontal sinus outlines is normal, but less than that often observed; the asymmetry of the maxillary sinuses is due to a fluid level in the R sinus, as a result of acute sinusitis.

panoramic images (see Chapter 2); conversely, the enamel margin at the cervical region of the tooth is not clearly delineated except mesially and distally, as the thin edge of enamel results in poor subject contrast.

(a) Continuity

The margins of teeth, and other hard tissue or soft tissue structures, should be followed in order to detect any break in continuity, which will either be indicative of a real change (which should be investigated and identified), or due to imaging problems. Examples of the former are the interrupted enamel surface due to an underlying carious lesion (Fig. 3.11a), the discontinuity in the cortical bone due to a fracture (Fig. 3.11b), and the local cessation of the margin of the ID canal due to close proximity to third molar apices (Fig. 3.12). An example of an imaging cause of discontinuity is the step in the lower border of the mandible, seen in panoramic views, due to patient movement during the exposure (Fig. 3.13a).

(b) Width

The radiographic width of any feature is determined by its real dimensions, and the projection geometry.

On the foundation of expected width, recognition of any alteration can be made:

(i) *Reduction in width.* This may be localized or generalized. If the variation is localized then it is often due to proximity with another feature, normal (Fig. 3.22a) or pathological (e.g. resulting from pressure of an expanding cyst, or destruction by an aggressive tumour); when generalized, the explanation may be due to a systemic disorder, or physiological age change (e.g. the progressive loss of height of alveolar bone in edentulous jaws) (Fig. 3.14).

(ii) *Increase in width.* An increase in width is often a response by tissue to some adjacent feature recognized as abnormal, and represents an attempt to wall off or enclose the abnormality (Fig. 3.15).

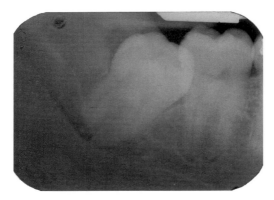

Fig. 3.12 Discontinuity of the upper border of the ID canal, associated with a slight downward deviation of the canal, and the apices of 48, indicates an intimate relationship between the apices and the canal: M 25.

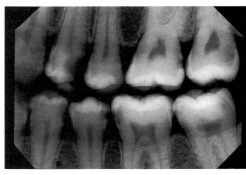

(a)

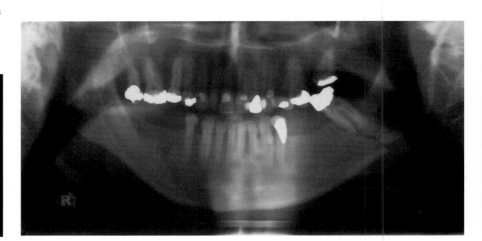

(b)

Fig. 3.11
(a) Caries evident on multiple surfaces: at the enamel surface there is a break in continuity, even when there is no cavitation.
(b) Fractured left body of mandible, resulting from a fall from a ladder; the appearance of the left condyle is peculiar due to superimposition of the anterior arch of the atlas (C1): M 40.

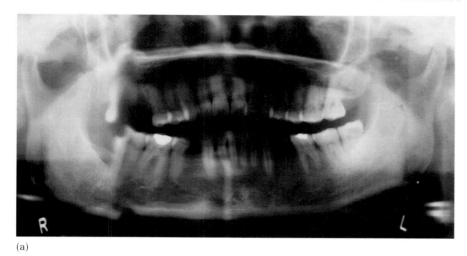

(a)

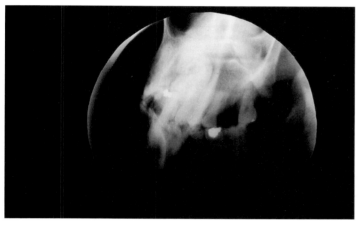

(b)

Fig. 3.13
(a) The discontinuity of the lower border of the R body of the mandible is not the only abnormality; the posterior teeth have an unusual appearance caused by patient movement during the exposure: F 53.
(b) There is no discontinuity on the oblique lateral view taken on the same visit.

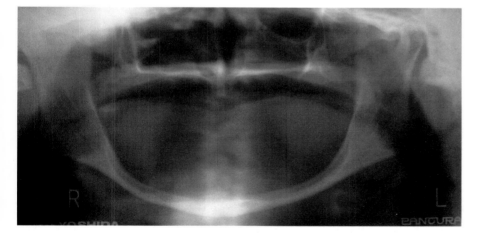

Fig. 3.14 Severely atrophied edentulous mandible; note the superficial ID canals and the surface position of the mental foramina: F 69.

3.3.8 Bone consistency

The pattern exhibited by cancellous bone in radiographs results from the arrangement of trabeculae, and is influenced by the exposure conditions. Alterations in the pattern occur in response to local and systemic factors, but there is surprisingly little change resulting from time alone.

The actual arrangement of the trabeculae shows wide variation within the limits of normal, and generally a similar pattern throughout a bone is indicative of normality. The exception to this rule is in situations where there is a systemic condition influencing the quality of the skeleton as a whole, such as osteoporosis, but knowledge of the patient's circumstances will alert the practitioner to this situation.

Local variation can be manifested as an increase or a decrease in the denseness of the trabecular pattern, which can be influenced by the loading on the bone; less variation is therefore seen in the ramus compared with the body of the mandible. The pattern exhibited can mimic pathological change, particularly when it is caused by a sparsity of trabeculae (Fig. 3.16).

3.3.9   Dentition

Leaving the examination of the teeth until this point should ensure that presence of an abnormality remote from the dentition has already been noted, and is unlikely to be overlooked, when the detailed treatment planning that arises from examination of the dentition takes place. It is helpful to consider four different aspects of the dentition:

(a) Number of teeth
(b) Eruption status
(c) Morphology
(d) Condition

(a) Number

Count the teeth. Knowledge of the number of teeth present can only be gained by identifying each tooth, erupted and unerupted. A hurried look at either a patient's mouth or the radiograph can result in errors: briefly glance at the radiograph in Fig. 3.17, decide on the impression as to which teeth are present, and then study it more carefully. The impression gained from intact rows of teeth is that there is a complete dentition; counting the teeth verifies or contradicts this impression.

The deciduous dentition consists of 20 teeth, and the permanent dentition of 32 teeth. They are arranged in groups according to function.

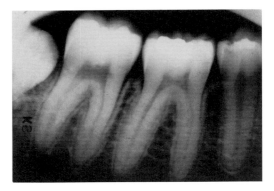

Fig. 3.16 Sparse trabecular pattern creating radiolucent 'areas'; the 'area' related to 47 distal apex is not pathological: the lamina dura is intact around the apex: M 17.

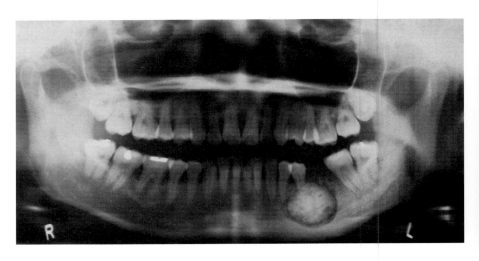

Fig. 3.15 Localized thickening of the lower cortical margin of the mandible, in relation to the obvious pathological lesion: F 29. (See also Fig. 3.29 and Fig. 9.11.)

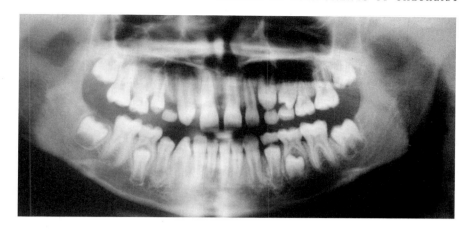

Fig. 3.17 The arches appear unbroken, but counting the teeth present, erupted and unerupted, reveals that the following permanent teeth are congenitally absent: 15, 12, 25: M 9.

(i) *Deciduous*

In each jaw:	incisors — four
	canines — two
	molars — four

FDI notation

	55 54 53 52 51	61 62 63 64 65	
Right			Left
	85 84 83 82 81	71 72 73 74 75	

(ii) *Permanent*

In each jaw:	incisors — four
	canines — two
	premolars — four
	molars — six

FDI notation

18 17 16 15 14 13 12 11	21 22 23 24 25 26 27 28	
Right		Left
48 47 46 45 44 43 42 41	31 32 33 34 35 36 37 38	

The permanent molars are the only teeth which do not have deciduous predecessors.

The FDI notation will be used throughout this book to identify individual teeth.

(iii) *Abnormalities of number.* Both supernumerary teeth (Fig. 3.18) and congenitally absent teeth are relatively common (Figs 3.17 and 3.19); these two conditions have a tendency to affect particular teeth, as do abnormalities of form if the teeth are present.

The teeth most frequently found to be congenitally absent are the third molar, the (upper) lateral incisor, and the (lower) second premolar. One explanation for this is found in the sequence of development of the teeth, and the natural groups that exist.

The eight teeth in each quadrant can be subdivided into three groups:

| Incisors | Cuspids | Molars |
| 1 2 | 3 4 5 | 6 7 8 |

The lateral incisor, second premolar, and third molar are each the last of a series and commence their development last within the group. Conversely, the first of each series: the central incisor, canine, and first molar, are generally the teeth least likely to be affected by developmental disorders in the permanent dentition. As with many 'generalizations' there are exceptions to the rule, and when lower incisors are congenitally absent it is not uncommon for them to be centrals rather than laterals.

(b) *Eruption status*
Note the eruption status of the teeth, and make a decision on whether it is normal. Unerupted or partially erupted teeth that may require removal should be examined with care and the following points noted for each:

(i)   state of eruption: unerupted or partially erupted;
(ii)   for unerupted teeth, the bony covering: complete or incomplete;
(iii)   angulation: vertical (normal or inverted orientation); mesial; distal; horizontal; transverse. If the tooth is transverse to the arch then a second radiograph will be necessary to determine which way the crown is facing, if it is intended to remove the tooth (see Chapter 4, Fig. 4.6).

(c) *Morphology*
Only certain external morphological features of the crown are routinely visible, such as the number and shape of cusps. In some situations the root surface may also be visible. Normally, however, features affecting other aspects of the tooth will only be evident from radiographs.

Box 3.1

Morphology = the study of the forms of things (Greek derivation, *morphe*, form, + -logy, a subject of study or interest).

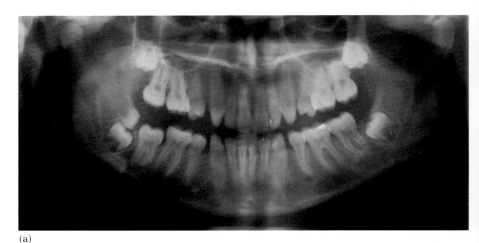

(a)

Fig. 3.18
(a) A supplemental third molar (49) is present in a position causing impaction of developing 48; the size of the molars progressively decreases from the first; the first premolars have been extracted for orthodontic reasons: F 14.
(b) Multiple supplemental premolars developing; they are at a much earlier stage of development than the normal series of permanent teeth: F 13.

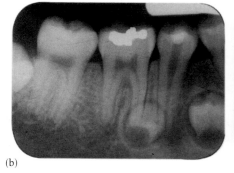 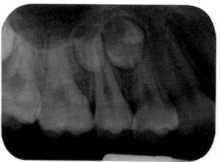

(b)

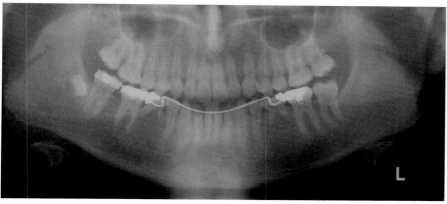

(a)

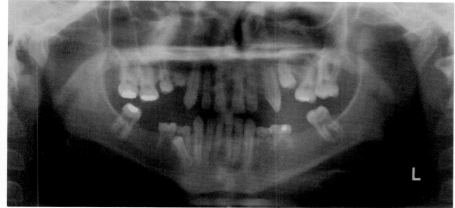

(b)

Fig. 3.19
(a) Congenitally absent 35 and 45, with the unusual appearance of a developing third molar in one of the affected quadrants; the second deciduous molars 75 and 85 are retained and are being used to assist in achieving a good arch form: M 14.
(b) Multiple congenitally absent teeth; the situation appears particularly severe due to early loss of 36 and 46 as a result of caries, which is also clearly evident in 37: M 15.

Recognition of morphological variations is dependent on knowledge, expectation, and visual acuity. The most straightforward way to detect morphological variations is to examine individual crowns as the teeth are counted, and then individual roots as the bone supporting the teeth is examined. Variations that are readily detectable on radiographs include variations in form and size of the pulp chamber, enamel invaginations, enamel evaginations, individual hypoplastic teeth, additional roots, and abnormalities of shape of roots. Any more widespread abnormality will also be evident but will normally have been detected by direct examination of the teeth. Figure 3.20 includes a selection of morphological abnormalities, and others are included in Chapters 5 and 6.

(d) *Condition*
The condition of the crowns of the teeth is dealt with in detail in Chapter 5.

3.3.10 Supporting bone

The important aspects of the supporting bone of the teeth, in respect of changes resulting from periodontal, pulpal, and other disorders is dealt with in detail in Chapter 7.

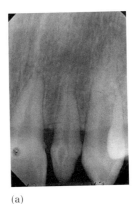
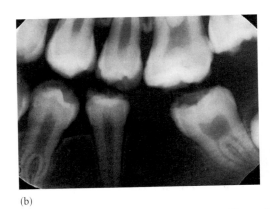
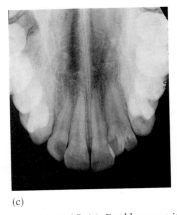

(a)   (b)   (c)

Fig. 3.20   (a) Conical-shaped upper lateral incisor, with invaginated enamel: F 20. (b) Bifid roots of lower first premolar: M 15. (c) Double crown in upper lateral incisor: M 12.

3.3.11   Any other features

This is often the most interesting part of examining radiographs — analysing the appearance caused by something out of the ordinary, that does not fall immediately into one of the common dental diseases. The feature(s) will have been picked up at an earlier point in the examination, and then left until the routine matters have been concluded: this reduces the risk of forgetting the routine elements of the complete sequence.

The notes in this section are brief and highlight the key significance of each of the features to be described. The chapters on radiolucent lesions (Chapter 8) and radiopaque and mixed lesions (Chapter 9) provide examples of a variety of disorders, with more extensive detail.

(a)   Radiolucent/radiopaque/combination
(b)   Site
(c)   Shape
(d)   Size
(e)   Margins
(f)   Relation to other structures (?aetiological factors)
(g)   Effect on other structures
(h)   Provisional/differential diagnosis

(a) Radiolucent/radiopaque/combination
The appearance of any feature on a radiograph, in terms of its degree of blackness or whiteness, is a useful pointer to its nature. Variations from the expected appearance trigger the need to determine an explanation.

The term 'radiolucent' is used to describe a feature that is relatively black in a radiographic image (i.e. the X-rays have been able to pass through the feature). This may be absolute or relative; an apparent 'radiolucency' may be due to an adjacent increased radiopacity.

Air is the most radiolucent normal feature, and its presence is indicated by the interface with structures delineating air spaces; abnormal presence of air within soft tissues is depicted as a radiolucency. Radiolucent abnormalities within otherwise hard tissues result from:

— a decrease in mineralization;
— a decrease in thickness; or
— a combination of the two;
— artefacts due to sensitization of the emulsion (e.g. pressure marks) (Fig. 3.21)

X-ray imaging is very sensitive to even relatively small differences in atomic structure of tissues and other materials. Absorption of X-ray photon energy is dependent on the photoelectric absorption effect (Chapter 1, p. 8). The probability of this occurring is proportional to the cube of the atomic number of the material in question. Examining the atomic numbers of bone and soft tissue explains why soft tissues are relatively radiolucent with respect to bone, and any alteration in the mineral content or quantity of bone will result in an alteration in the degree of radiolucency or radiopacity.

Bone, average atomic number, $Z = 12$; 12 cubed $= 1728$
Soft tissue, average atomic number, $Z = 7$; 7 cubed $= 343$

Thus, the probability of the X-ray beam undergoing attenuation by absorption is much greater in bone than in soft tissue.

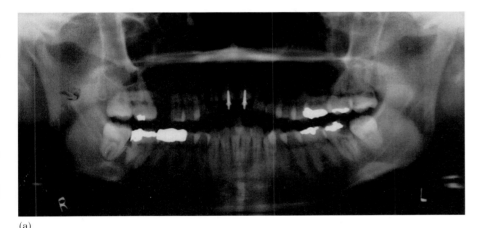

(a)

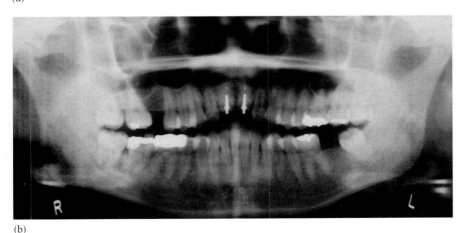

(b)

Fig. 3.21
(a) Unusual radiolucency apparently in the right ramus, resulting from pressure marks, due to poor handling: F 29.
(b) A repeat film demonstrates there is no abnormality.

The term 'radiopacity' is used to describe a feature that is relatively white on a radiograph. Radiopaque images are evident within both hard and soft tissues and result from normal structures, and abnormalities, due to:

— an increase in mineralization (e.g. sclerosing osteitis, depicting chronic inflammatory changes in bone).
— an increase in thickness of a structure in the path of the X-ray beam (e.g. caused by a change in the relation between the object and the X-ray beam, Fig. 3.22a).
— superimposition of two normal features (e.g. overlapping enamel, Fig. 3.22b).
— a calcified component of soft tissue (e.g. calcified lymph nodes).
— anything replacing air in the maxillary sinus (e.g. a mucous retention cyst, Fig. 3.23).
— certain foreign bodies, or restorations (e.g. metal and other opaque restorations).
— artefacts (e.g. an opacity on an extra-oral radiograph caused by light being prevented from reaching the film: dust on the intensifying screens commonly results in this problem, Fig. 3.24).

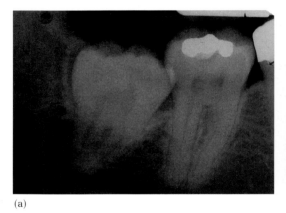

(a)

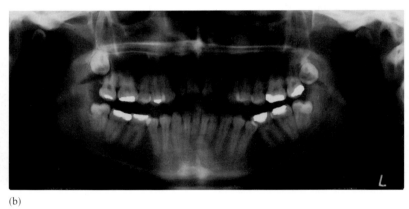

(b)

Fig. 3.22
(a) The root mass of 48 is dilacerated, so that the apices are in line with the X-ray beam and appear locally more radiopaque; the ID canal is locally narrowed, indicating a very close relationship with the apices: F 28.
(b) Due to crowding the images of 35 and 45 are overlapped with the images of 36 and 46; the increased quantity of enamel in the path of the X-ray beam causes an increase in radiopacity. Note also the appearance of the crowns of 18 and 28 which are obliquely transverse to the arch, altering the enamel component that is demonstrated in the image: F 26.

Fig. 3.23 F, 12 in mixed dentition stage with full complement of teeth: 23 is erupting mesially and causing resorption of the apices of 21 and 22; examination of the upper right quadrant indicates that the path of eruption of 13 caused similar resorption of 12. Gross caries is evident in the deciduous molars. In addition to these dental findings there is a domed radiopacity in the left maxillary sinus typical of a mucous retention cyst — this illustrates the influence of the surrounding medium on the radiolucency or radiopacity of a feature; in this situation replacing the normal radiolucent air with any other material will result in the lesion acquiring a radiopaque appearance. (See also Fig. 3.9: a lateral cephalometric radiograph which provides confirmation of position of crown of 23 in same plane as roots of 21 and 22.)

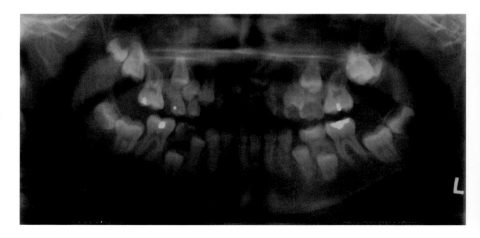

(b) *Site*

Identifying the site or sites in which a lesion is situated is important in considering the possible aetiology. The following sites can be used:

- Dental
  — coronal
  — radicular

- Alveolar (in the mandible this is specifically above the inferior dental canal)
  — pericoronal
  — periradicular
  — periapical
- Basal: not directly related to teeth
- Bones other than the maxilla and mandible
- Extra-osseous

The site of a lesion is often linked firmly with possible aetiological factors. A common example of this is a periapical lesion; a lesion described as periapical is more likely to have resulted from a problem related to components of the tooth than from another cause (e.g. a periapical inflammatory lesion resulting from a non-vital pulp). The other sites and their influence on diagnosis, are referred to predominantly in later chapters; definitions of the various sites is covered in Box 3.3.

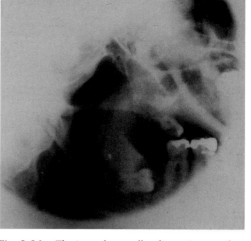

Fig. 3.24 The irregular small radiopacity near the lingula and above the upper border of the ID canal is caused by dust inside the cassette, preventing light from reaching the film. There is an increase in size and loss of definition of the follicular space associated with 48 (see Fig. 8.5 and Fig. 9.18): M 54

Box 3.3

periapical: peri = round, about; apex = a tip or pointed end (plural — apexes or apices).
coronal = circlet for the head (of a tooth).
radicular: radical = of the roots.
alveolar = of an alveolus: alveolus = the bony socket for the root of a tooth.
basal = of, at, or forming a base.
osseous = consisting of bone, ossified.

One of the most important conclusions that can result from accurately describing the site of a lesion is whether or not it may be of odontogenic origin. Any lesion affecting a tooth or within the alveolar bone and having a clear relationship to a tooth, or the site where a tooth has been, may be odon-

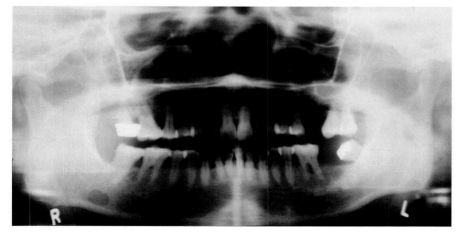

Fig. 3.25 Oval radiolucency near the right angle of the mandible must be non-odontogenic in origin; Stafne cavity: F 50. (See also Fig. 8.29.)

togenic in origin. Conversely, a lesion that is entirely within the basal bone of the mandible, as delineated by the inferior dental canal, cannot be odontogenic in origin (Fig. 3.25), unless the lesion has powers of migration: in practice only teeth have this ability (Fig. 3.26). A number of pathological odontogenic lesions may present predominantly outside the alveolar portion of the jaws due to expansion.

(c) Shape

The shape of a lesion can provide information about its pattern of growth, which may be regular or irregular. Some common descriptive terms are widely used:

(i) *Round*, signifying even expansion: a lesion that is round on a single radiograph will probably also be round in the third dimension, and can be thought of as expanding like a balloon being inflated.

(ii) *Oval*: an oval shape is frequently a modification of round, and results from the influence on a lesion of different adjacent features. A good example of this is the differing influence of cancellous and cortical bone. An expanding lesion is likely to have its shape influenced by cortical bone, due to the greater resistance to resorption that it exerts, as compared to cancellous bone which is relatively easily resorbed, being less uniform in nature.

The even growth and expansion indicated by both circular and oval lesions indicates that such lesions have a high probability of being benign, particularly when there is a clear aetiological factor. The lack of an aetiological factor should raise an element of doubt, as there is a very important exception to the general rule: both the solitary plasmacytoma and multiple myeloma are depicted on radiographs as circular radiolucencies.

(i) *Scalloped* (small rounded lobes): round and oval shapes can be modified by a scalloping effect at the margin; this is suggestive of irregular growth as caused by certain pathological lesions (e.g. the odontogenic keratocyst).

(ii) *Irregular*: a completely irregular shape which does not suggest a descriptive label is more likely to be caused by an aggressive inflammatory or malignant lesion, which has an infiltrative, rather than expanding, nature of growth.

Examples of pathological lesions exhibiting varying appearances can be found throughout the text, and particularly in Chapters 8 and 9.

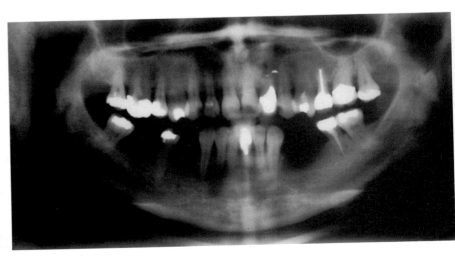

Fig. 3.26 A premolar has migrated into the left ramus; the root is not clear due to its position relative to the plane in focus: F 42.

(d) Size

The size of a lesion on its own is not very useful, as both benign and malignant lesions may present radiologically when small or large. Other features need to be considered in conjunction with the size which may give an indication of the probable time frame, for example, a large lesion with a well-defined margin is likely to be a benign lesion which has been present for a considerable time (months or even years). Conversely, a large lesion whose margins are difficult to detect is more likely to be a lesion undergoing rapid change.

A few radiological features have a characteristic size, for example, the early sign of a developing tooth prior to any evidence of calcification has a similar size regardless of which precise tooth it is, but dependent on the form of the tooth: incisor, canine, premolar, or molar, normal series or supernumerary (Fig. 3.27).

(e) Margins

The margins of a lesion can be described in two ways, well defined and ill defined:

(i) *Well defined*: there is a clear distinction between abnormal and normal. This is indicative of a contained lesion, most probably benign (Fig. 3.28).

In addition to this clear definition some radiolucent lesions have a white line around them, representing cortication, caused by a reaction of the surrounding bone to low-grade stimulus. This is only seen with benign, uninfected lesions (e.g. a radicular cyst, Fig. 3.28). The corollary to this sometimes seen in conjunction with radiopaque lesions is a surrounding radiolucent zone, which indicates a soft tissue separation zone between the lesion and the bone (Fig. 3.29).

(ii) *Ill defined*: this is suggestive of infiltration due to aggressive inflammatory change or malignancy (Fig. 3.30). The observation of an ill-defined margin is one of the key features that should alert the dentist to the need to investigate a lesion urgently.

(f) Relation to other structures (?aetiological factors)

The need to consider the possible aetiology of a lesion has already been mentioned. One of the most helpful features in this context is the precise relationship that the lesion has with other structures, for example, a radiolucency

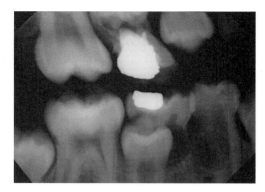

Fig. 3.27 Superimposed on the root of 44 is a radiolucency depicting the crypt of a forming supernumerary tooth germ; mineralization is just commencing: M 10

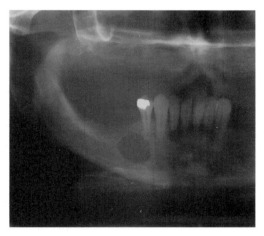

Fig. 3.28 The periapical radiolucency associated with 42 is well defined, but does not have a corticated margin; the larger radiolucency in the right body of the mandible is well defined, and corticated, indicating that growth is slow and there is little inflammation at present: M 33. (See Fig. 8.7.)

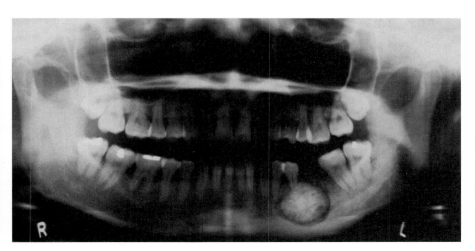

Fig. 3.29 The striking, mainly radiopaque, lesion in the left body of the mandible is surrounded by a radiolucent zone, indicating a soft tissue separation zone between the lesion and the surrounding bone. The lower border of the mandible is thicker in this region indicating long-standing low-grade chronic inflammation, and an attempt by the cortex to enclose the abnormality: F 29. (See Fig. 9.11.)

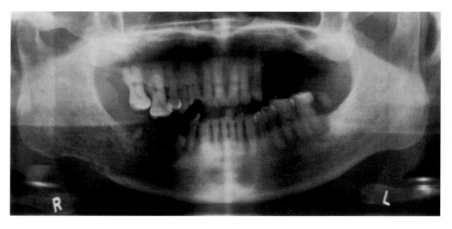

Fig. 3.30 There is a patchy, destructive lesion in the right body and ramus of the mandible with margins that are ill defined, with a pathological fracture through the lower border of the mandible; this malignant lesion was a metastasis from a primary adenocarcinoma of the prostate; note the marked attrition affecting a number of teeth, caries, and exfoliation of the remaining root of 38: M 82.

completely enclosing the crown of an unerupted tooth has a considerable chance of having arisen from the dental follicle (reduced enamel epithelium), and being a dentigerous cyst.

(g) Effect on other structures

A lesion, when small, is likely to have no effect on other structures. As a lesion increases in size, there are five possible findings, which may occur sequentially, and are well demonstrated elsewhere in the text:

(i) *No effect*: the lesion adapts to existing structures without altering them in any way (e.g. solitary bone cysts, until relatively large when expansion of the overlying bone may occur).

(ii) *Displacement*: displacement of teeth or of the inferior dental canal, usually indicates a slow, benign growth (e.g. most cysts, fibrous dysplasia, giant cell granuloma). Displacement of unaltered structures requires the initiation of bone resorption and deposition; this is normally a physiological process and cannot be accelerated. This is well known when applying orthodontic forces to move teeth; attempts to speed up the process by increasing the force results in the teeth coming to a stop.

(iii) *Expansion*: expansion of cortical bone occurs in a manner similar to displacement of other anatomical structures, and is most commonly associated with relatively benign lesions; early expansion may be superseded by destruction as the lesion increases in size.

(iv) *Resorption*: resorption of both teeth and bone needs osteoclasts, and time. It is a feature that is generally related to benign but aggressive lesions (e.g. ameloblastoma), and is also seen in inflammatory lesions where release of osteoclast-activating factor is a common component of the pathological process.

(v) *Aggressive destruction*: fast-growing aggressive lesions, which destroy the bone supporting the teeth, can cause marked displacement of teeth by effectively carrying them on the edge of the expanding lesion. In this situation the normal supporting structures are lost, and frequently also the relationship with adjacent teeth.

(h) Provisional/differential diagnosis

This final step in the description of a lesion is the reason for going through the other stages, and is the most important step in deciding the best approach to patient management. There are daily situations where a decision about the diagnosis can be made apparently without much thought, as with classical carious lesions. There are also times when the initial reaction is: 'I have no idea what this is'. In such a situation a careful description and assessment of the information provided by the descriptive status can change confusion into a structured and appropriate plan of action.

A provisional diagnosis is a single diagnosis, which is indicated by the combination of findings to be the most likely diagnosis. It is unusual in radiology to be more positive than this although there are exceptions, for example, the firm diagnosis of a Stafne cavity (Fig. 3.25) is made for radiolucent lesions fulfilling the following criteria: radiolucent; beneath the inferior dental canal; near the angle of the mandible; round or oval; well-defined, corticated margin; not related to other structures; having no effect on other structures; and causing no symptoms. This last point concerning the absence of symptoms is important, and if there is any doubt about the diagnosis then the lesion must be reviewed radiographically, after six to twelve months.

A differential diagnosis is a list of possible diagnoses, on the basis of the information so far available. It is customary to list the conditions in descending order of likelihood, although the possibility of malignancy should be included early in the list to ensure that it is investigated fully, and at an early stage.

A useful *aide-mémoire* to assist in focusing the information gleaned from the available radiographs, together with clinical information, is a radiological sieve. This is based on the widely used surgical sieve, an approach to categorizing all possible situations:

Radiological sieve

- Normal
- Developmental
- Traumatic
- Inflammatory
- Cystic
- Neoplastic
- Osteodystrophy
- Metabolic/systemic
- Idiopathic
- Iatrogenic
- Foreign body
- Artefact

This list can be used as a checklist against the features of a lesion, in order to highlight areas requiring in-depth consideration. The question can be asked: 'could it be ... normal, inflammatory, etc.?' A positive 'no' eliminates that possibility resulting in a shorter list of possibilities to deal with. In order to eliminate still further it may be necessary to carry out other investigations, and these will be covered under the section on proposals in this chapter.

3.3.12   Summary

It is important to summarize the main radiological findings in order to clarify their relative importance, and ensure that nothing has been missed. A brief summary can be incorporated in the patient's clinical notes as a report, and to assist in checking that appropriate treatment has been carried out. The description of the lesions illustrated in Chapters 8 and 9 is provided in the form of a summary, linking the individual features.

3.3.13   Proposals to meet patient's requirements, including other investigations

The radiographic examination and interpretation is one step in the overall process of providing treatment for a patient. The views to be taken will be determined by the clinical examination. The next stage in a patient's investigation, or treatment, often results from proposals made as a result of the radiological findings. An example that occurs quite frequently is the discovery of a periapical radiolucency. A rapid response to this is to assume that the tooth is non-vital, and plan to commence endodontic therapy. However, there are other situations that can cause such radiolucencies, including normal anatomical features (see Fig. 3.16 and Chapters 2 and 8), and pathological lesions which are not secondary to pulpal death (Chapters 8 and 9). In view of this, a logical proposal would be to carry out a sensitivity test on the tooth before commencing any radical treatment.

Potential further investigations that might be indicated as a result of the radiographic examination are:

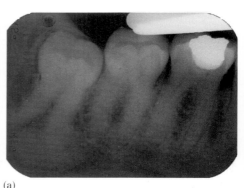

(a)

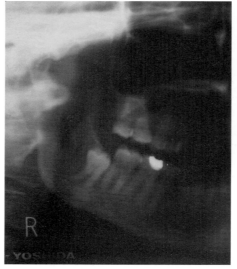

(a)

Fig. 3.31
(a) Radiographic investigation of impacted third molars revealed a radiopaque mass related to the mesial apex of deeply impacted 48; the opacity is well circumscribed and appears to be continuous with the mesial root; asymptomatic: F 47. A differential diagnosis of cementoma; idiopathic osteosclerosis was made, and radiographic review planned.
(b) 7 months later there is no discernible change in the radiopacity; no further treatment is indicated.

(b)

- Clinical tests
- Biopsy
- Further conventional radiography
- CT (computed tomography), and/or
- Other specialized imaging techniques (e.g. ultrasound, radioisotope imaging, MRI (magnetic resonance imaging))

Brief notes on specialized imaging techniques, with illustrations, are provided in Appendix D.

Review

There are many situations where there is no firm indication for urgent action, but a question mark still hangs over the final diagnosis. In situations like this, and only if there is no possibility of malignancy, radiographic review, using the same technique to provide comparative images, is often the wisest course (Fig. 3.31). Such a review should allow time for possible changes to occur, so that a difference in appearance is detectable. Suitable periods will range from three to twelve months, dependent on individual circumstances.

3.4 APPLICATIONS

A number of examples have been used in this chapter to illustrate specific points. The application of the *system of examination* to lesions that are suspected of being abnormalities, is covered more fully in Chapters 8 and 9, which deal specifically with lesions that present with a radiolucent,

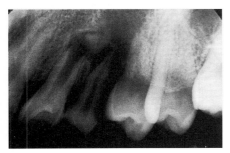

(b)

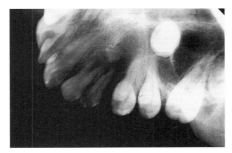

(c)

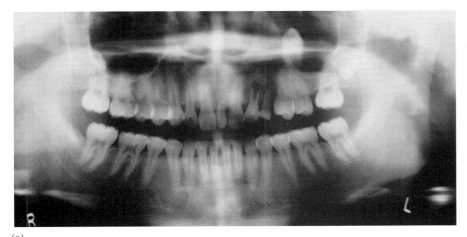

(a)

Fig. 3.32

(a) Panoramic radiograph of M, 17 with retained 63 and no sign of 23 in the mouth; erupted mesiodens between 11 and 21; no clinical caries or other findings of note (Chinese teenager brought up in fluoridated area). 23 is present, inverted with its apex superimposed on the apices of 24/25; 63 is associated with a periapical area of radiolucency also involving the adjacent 22, which has an open apex.
(b) The periapical view clearly shows the enamel invagination in 22 that is implicated in its early loss of vitality approximately 18 months after eruption; there is some opacity within the area of bone resorption, possibly representing calcium deposition in granulation tissue.
(c) The oblique occlusal centred on the premolars enables accurate localization of 23 with respect to the arch, and assessment of its orientation, by means of vertical parallax; the tooth is seen in cross-section indicating that it is aligned to the path of the X-ray beam with its crown more buccal than its apex; the apex is palatal to the premolar apices.

radiopaque, or mixed appearance. In particular, some of the examples used in this chapter to illustrate specific points are dealt with more fully.

The case illustrated on the front cover demonstrates the value of a thorough examination of all parts of the radiographic image, and combining the information provided by different views (Fig. 3.32). Reference to details of radiographic and localization techniques will supplement the caption information.

4 Localization using dental radiography

4.1	INTRODUCTION	70
	4.1.1 Radiographic localization	**70**
4.2	VIEWING RADIOGRAPHS	71
4.3	VIEWS AT RIGHT-ANGLES	72
4.4	PARALLAX	74
	4.4.1 Definition	**75**
	4.4.2 Visual application	**75**
	4.4.3 Radiographic application	**76**
4.5	USEFUL RADIOGRAPHIC COMBINATIONS	80
	4.5.1 Periapicals	**80**
	4.5.2 Bitewings	**81**
	4.5.3 Occlusals	**82**
	4.5.4 Combinations of different projections	**82**
4.6	POOR COMBINATIONS	85
4.7	RADIOPAQUE MARKERS	86
4.8	SELF-ASSESSMENT EXAMPLES	87
4.9	ANSWERS TO SELF-ASSESSMENT EXAMPLES	87

4 Localization using dental radiography

When dealing with more than one item at the same time, whether they are similar or quite different, they must have an intrinsic relationship to each other. Having some background knowledge that relates to these items makes it easier to consider what that relationship might be, and then to verify it. This is illustrated by the method used to arrange books in a library: books are usually classified by subject, and within that subject by author. With an understanding of this concept it is usually fairly straightforward to find any one particular book. This type of exercise is influenced by an academic knowledge of the subject matter, and also the ability to read: someone who knows nothing about medical or dental subjects will be at a disadvantage in a specialized library, as would someone who could not read. Two things are therefore needed in order to determine the relationship of items to each other, and these can be thought of as knowledge and application.

This chapter will:

1. Highlight the relevance of an awareness of the relationships of structures.
2. Clarify the role that dental radiography plays in establishing the relationship.
3. Provide a variety of examples to establish the reader's confidence.

4.1.1 Radiographic localization

Caries and periodontal disease provide two common everyday examples to justify the application of dental radiography (radiographic localization) in localization.

1. Caries can occur on all coronal and cervical surfaces, which are traditionally examined visually together, at times, with tactile methods to determine which surface is affected, and the extent of the lesion. Only lesions causing macroscopic surface changes can be detected in this manner. The depth cannot be accurately determined and therefore the relationship with the pulpal tissues is unknown.

2. The location of sites in the alveolar margin affected by destructive periodontal disease is made possible by tactile (instrumental) methods; direct vision is of limited value due to the presence of overlying soft tissue.

Many disorders affecting the crowns of teeth can also be assessed using visual and tactile methods, but beyond that there is a restrictive barrier created by the supporting structures of the dentition. Radiography assists in seeing through many of these barriers, and enhances the ability to determine relevant structural relationships.

Radiological sieve approach

All aspects of dentistry involve a knowledge of the relationship of individual objects to each other. There are innumerable situations where this is critical to both treatment planning, and provision of appropriate treatment. This section clarifies this need by indicating examples within each of the categories of the 'radiological sieve', (Chapter 3, p. 65), where radiographic localization is an advantage, and is likely to influence diagnosis and treatment planning:

Anatomical (normal): the precise location of normal anatomical features, such as air cavities, foramina, and neurovascular channels; the relation of teeth to each other and to such anatomical features.

Developmental (normal and abnormal): the location and orientation of unerupted normal and supernumerary teeth, and identification of anomalies within individual teeth.

Traumatic: the orientation of fracture lines in both teeth and jaws influences displacement of the fragments, and the suitable treatment options.

Inflammatory: lesions affecting dental and supporting tissues, such as caries, periodontal, and periapical lesions. Endodontic treatment is a common sequel to inflammatory disorders affecting the dental pulp, and demands accurate distinction of separate pulp canals.

Cystic: these lesions may be odontogenic or non-odontogenic in origin. Their position and relationship assists in determining an appropriate differential diagnosis.

Neoplastic: both benign and malignant lesions can become quite extensive. Small or large, their relationship with adjacent structures assists in both diagnosis and recognizing factors which will influence treatment options.

Osteodystrophies: disorders, such as fibrous dysplasia, can cause deformities, and impinge on other structures.

Metabolic/systemic: the extent of such disorders brings in the question of involvement of other bones and tissues.

Idiopathic: the location and relations of some radiologically evident entities is the key to their diagnosis. The Stafne idiopathic bone cavity is an excellent example (Fig. 3.25).

Iatrogenic: problems attributable to dental treatment are labelled iatrogenic; their recognition is aided by a full knowledge of previous treatment, in conjunction with accurate localization.

Foreign bodies: in addition to obvious foreign bodies, arising external to the person, normal structures can occur in ectopic sites.

4.2   VIEWING RADIOGRAPHS

Normal convention is to view radiographs from the position of the tube; for bitewings, periapicals, and oblique occlusals this places the patient's right side to the examiner's left on the X-ray viewing box, divided into four quadrants by the occlusal plane and the midline of the face (Fig. 4.1). In order to simplify interpretation, particularly in applying the principles of parallax, all other

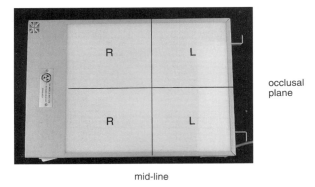

Fig. 4.1 Viewing box template.

radiographs are also viewed with the right and left sides of the patient conforming to the viewing box template.

The various cross-sectional or plan views do not readily fit into this system, and are arranged and viewed as follows:

Lower true occlusals and vertex occlusal: as from above, and as if standing in front of the patient;

Submentovertex (SMV):   as from below.

In each case the patient's right and left will then conform with other views.

Multiple views are best arranged on the viewing box to reflect their relationship with each other, thus indicating the difference in projection geometry in the horizontal, and/or vertical direction. In situations where the images in two views are expected to be very similar, incorporation of markers at the time of radiography can assist in their interpretation, although this is not necessary if different teeth are incorporated in the field of view.

Using radiographs for localization normally requires at least two views: a number of combinations of radiographs can be used to cause an apparent movement between objects that is fundamental to establishing their relationship. These are covered in the following sections. In each case, it is necessary to have an understanding of the geometrical principles involved in producing the various views (see Chapter 2).

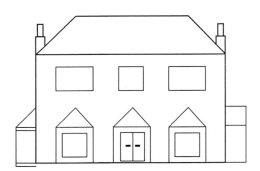

Fig. 4.2a Frontal elevation of a house.

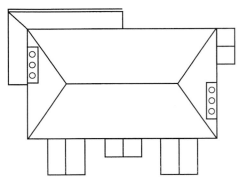

Fig. 4.2b Plan view of the same house.

4.3   VIEWS AT RIGHT-ANGLES

Views that are related to each other in this way enable two completely different perspectives of the same objects to be achieved. This is similar to the architect's elevation and plan views of a house (Fig. 4.2). In such a simplified example it is easy to appreciate how both views are needed to provide sufficient combined information to determine, for example: where the chimney are sited on the roof; whether the doorways and windows are flush with the building surface, set in or projecting outwards.

In the maxillo-facial region combinations of views at right angles are:

● Lateral and postero-anterior (PA) cephalometric radiographs.
● Lateral, PA, and submentovertex (SMV) skull or facial views.

- Panoramic, or paralleling periapical, and true mandibular occlusal views.
- Panoramic, or paralleling periapical, and vertex occlusal: the vertex occlusal has historically been used for localization, as it gives a plan view of the upper jaw (Fig. 4.3). Its use is not encouraged, as it results in a higher radiation dose to the patient, and can only be taken with an intensifying screen–film combination, within a special cassette.

The application of extra-oral views in this manner is illustrated in Fig. 4.4. The lateral view (Fig. 4.4a) enables antero-posterior and supero-inferior location of the object in question; the radiopaque object is superimposed on the upper second molars near to their apices. The PA view (Fig. 4.4b) is used to determine its lateral position, where it is seen to be superimposed on the ramus of the mandible — it must be remembered that the height of the object in this projection will be influenced by the extension–flexion position of the head, and its depth within the patient. Neither view is adequate on its own but combining the information in the two of them, it can be determined that the airgun pellet must be in the left cheek. Note the beaten silver appearance of the skull vault. This pattern of markings is typical of craniostenosis, a condition in which the skull sutures become obliterated, and the skull responds to pressure changes by resorption internally.

Two different dental examples are shown in Figs 4.5 and 4.6: the panoramic radiograph (Fig. 4.5a) shows a radiopacity in the region of the roots of 43 and 44. From this view alone it is not possible to deduce whether the opaque object is within the mandible, or a structure facial or lingual to it, attached or separate. The mandibular true occlusal (Fig. 4.5b) clearly demonstrates that it is lingual and separate. Applying the appropriate decision-making process enables a provisional or differential diagnosis to be formulated. The radiopacity in this case was due to a submandibular salivary gland calculus. The calculus is projected onto the image of the teeth at a higher level

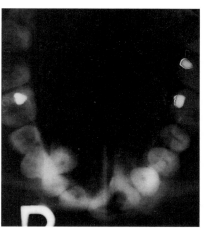

Fig. 4.3 Vertex occlusal radiograph taken with the central X-ray beam directed along the long axes of the upper incisors, resulting in a cross-sectional view of the teeth with clear radiolucencies depicting the pulp canals. The image of 13 can be seen palatal to the arch; the long axis of the tooth is parallel to the erupted teeth: M 22.

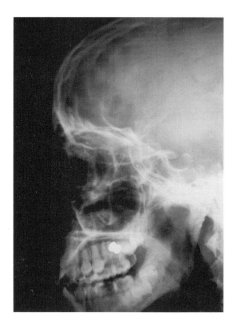

Fig. 4.4a An airgun pellet is seen as a clearly delineated, radiopaque object superimposed on the apices of the upper second molars; the height and antero-posterior position is obtained from this view.

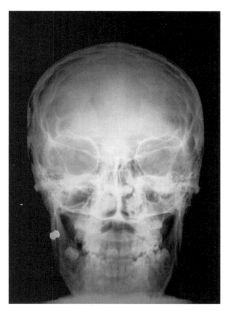

Fig. 4.4b In this PA view the lateral position is shown: it is superimposed on the ramus of the mandible. Reproduced with kind permission of Churchill-Livingstone.

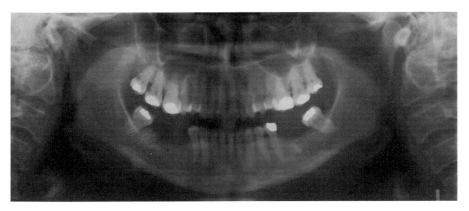

Fig. 4.5a   The radiopaque mass in the region of 44/43 could be within the mandible or superimposed: F 44.

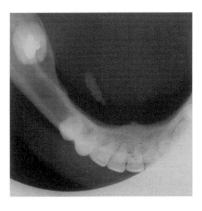

Fig. 4.5b   The true occlusal view clearly shows it is separate from the mandible.

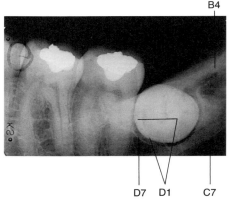

Fig. 4.6a   The impacted third molar is lying transverse to the dental arch; a surgical approach will be influenced by the buccal or lingual position of the crown: M 29.

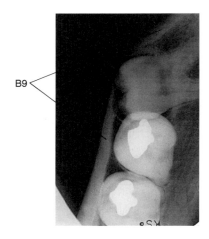

Fig. 4.6b   The true occlusal view, taken with a periapical film packet, clearly demonstrates the lingual position of the crown.

than expected, due to the upward direction of the X-ray beam in panoramic radiography, where the beam is transmitted from lingual to buccal, thus projecting a more lingual object higher than it is in reality.

It is important to note that the second radiograph may not always be necessary if the object of interest is palpable, or a clear history limits the possible locations to be considered. Figure 4.7 is a lateral neck view of a 13-year-old boy who knew he had lost a section of orthodontic arch wire from his mouth into his throat; the question to be answered was whether he had swallowed the fragment or was in danger of inhaling it. As there was no possibility of the wire being other than in the lumen or soft tissue of the alimentary canal or airway one view was sufficient.

4.4   PARALLAX

The shape of the jaws, the arrangement of teeth, and the proximity of other components of the cranio-facial skeleton limits the use of views at right-angles to each other. For all other combinations of radiographs an in-depth understanding of the principles of parallax enables accurate interpretation to be carried out.

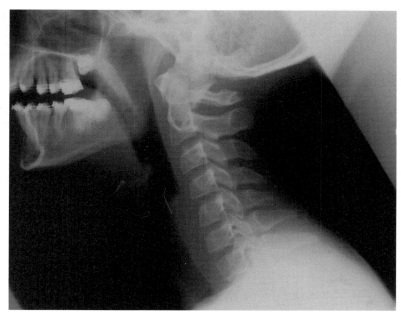

Fig. 4.7 An orthodontic wire which has been swallowed and become lodged in the larynx: M 13

4.4.1 Definition

Parallax

Apparent displacement, or difference in the apparent position, of an object, caused by an actual change (or difference) of position of the point of observation.

It is important to develop an understanding of just how the change in observation point determines the apparent change of position of the object of interest.

4.4.2 Visual application

Failing to locate an item because it is hidden by something else is a common occurrence. When a different vantage point is adopted from where objects do not overlap, their relative position becomes clear; the actual relationship of the objects in question has not altered in any way, only the observer's viewpoint.

Consider looking into a store cupboard containing a number of different items. Only the front ones can be properly identified (Fig. 4.8a), even though the presence of others may be indicated if they are taller or wider. It would be possible to move the items in question around in order to see them all, but it is quicker to look from a slightly different vantage point by moving one's head to a different position. It will then become clear what the objects are as they separate out from each other (Fig. 4.8b).

The further the observer's head is moved the more they will separate (Fig. 4.8c). The amount of apparent movement between the objects is dependent on their proximity to each other, in conjunction with the displacement of the observer's position; the direction of apparent movement is dependent on their relative position to the observer:

- objects very close to each other will not separate much regardless of the extent of change of the observer's position;
- the object furthest from the observer appears to move in the same direction as the observer;

- the object closest to the observer appears to move in the opposite direction to the observer; and
- objects between the two extremes adopt a position reflecting their place in the order from front to back.

A simple test using one's own fingers verifies this quickly and convincingly:

> Hold your hands in front of you at eye level each with one finger pointing straight up, hands held together so that the two fingers are superimposed (Fig. 4.9a). Now, without moving your hands; move your head to the left or right, the finger furthest from you will appear to move in the same direction as your head (Figs 4.9b and c). The same principle can be illustrated by moving in a vertical direction (Fig. 4.10).

From these examples it is clear that by knowing the direction of change in the observer's position, the apparent change in the object position can be accurately analysed.

4.4.3   Radiographic application

In radiography, the X-ray tube and the observer are equivalent to each other. The principle of parallax can be applied to interpretation, provided that the effective directional change in the position of the X-ray tube between two views is known, and the images are assessed according to that change. It is frequently not necessary to take special views — views that incorporate both the object to be localized and the same reference point can be used without exposing the patient to further radiation, even when taken on different dates, provided there has been little or no change in the real position of the object. Combinations that are of use are illustrated in this chapter, and reference made to combinations which are not useful.

The acronym, SLOB, is helpful in interpreting the radiographs, and applies to horizontal and vertical movements.

> *Interpretation of directional movement*
>
> S ame
> L ingual
> O pposite
> B uccal

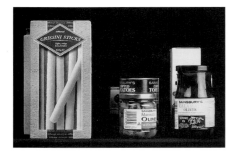

Fig. 4.8a   The objects at the back of the shelf are obscured by the front row, except where they are taller or wider.

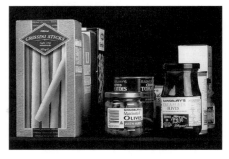

Fig. 4.8b   The observer has moved to the right causing the contents of the shelf to change in appearance: the objects to the back of the shelf have moved to the right of those at the front.

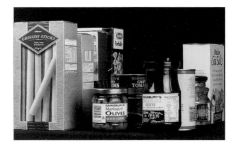

Fig. 4.8c   The observer has moved further to the right: the objects are separating out more than in Fig. 4.8b.

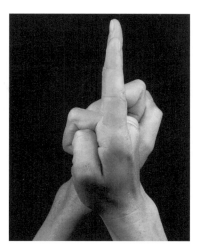

Fig. 4.10a   The eyes are at a higher level than the fingers; the furthest one is higher than the nearest.

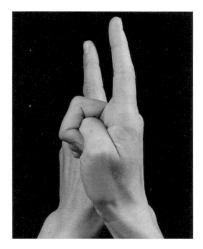

Fig. 4.9b   Moving the head to the left moves the furthest finger to the left.

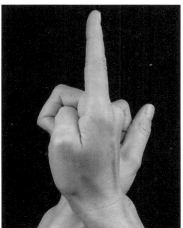

Fig. 4.9a   The two index fingers are superimposed.

Fig. 4.10b   The eyes are level with the fingers.

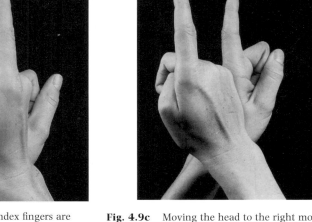

Fig. 4.9c   Moving the head to the right moves the furthest finger to the right.

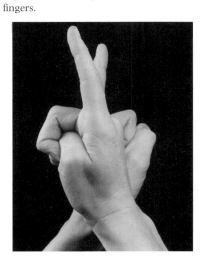

Fig. 4.10c   The eyes are at a lower level than the fingers; the nearest one has moved up in the opposite direction to the change of position of the eyes.

This acronym can be illustrated diagrammatically, and with equivalent radiographs (Figs 4.11 and 4.12).

A second acronym, BUILD, can be used in situations where the useful movement is vertical.

B uccal
U p
I
L ingual
D own

The addition of a single letter, I, to the initials BULD gives the world BUILD.

This can be illustrated diagrammatically (Fig. 4.13) using the relationship between the apices of an impacted lower third molar, and the inferior dental canal.

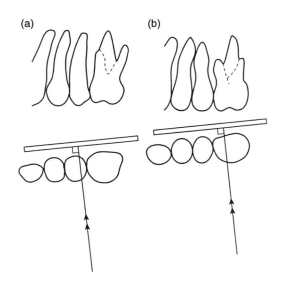

Fig. 4.11a   The central ray is directed at 90° to the arch through 25.
Fig. 4.11b   The tube has been shifted distally to direct the central ray through 26; the beam is still at 90° to the arch.

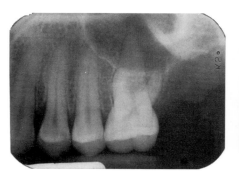

Fig. 4.12a   The central ray is directed at 90° to the arch through 25; the mesio-buccal root is superimposed on the palatal root.

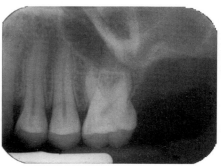

Fig.4 12b   The tube has been shifted distally to direct the central ray through 26; the beam is still at 90° to the arch; the mesio-buccal root has moved in the opposite direction so that all three roots can be clearly seen.

(a)

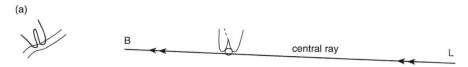

Fig.4 13a The X-ray beam in the panoramic projection passes through the mandible from lingual to buccal, at a slight upward angulation, but the radiograph is viewed as if from the buccal aspect; the apices of the third molar are superimposed on the image of the ID canal.

(b)

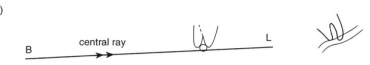

Fig. 4.13b The X-ray beam in the periapical passes from buccal to lingual, and at a deliberate slight upward angulation; one apex of the third molar has moved up (buccal), and the other down (lingual), relative to the ID canal.

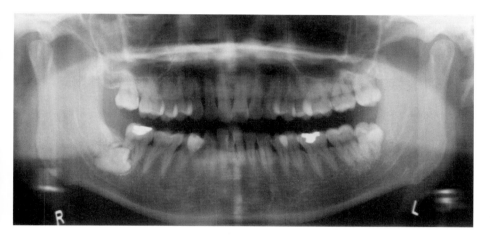

Fig. 4.14a A deeply impacted, horizontal lower right third molar; the crown is overlapping the distal root of 47 which can be seen as well, indicating that one is buccal to the other; the upper margin of 48 is 4 mm. below the alveolar ridge. The apices of 48 are closely related to the upper border of the ID canal: M 30.

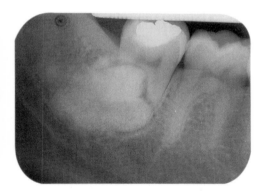

Fig. 4.14b The periapical view has projected the crown of 48 more mesial in relation to 47, and closer to the alveolar margin. Horizontal differences between panoramic and intra-oral radiographs are confusing and liable to lead to errors of judgement. The vertical difference is easier to interpret; movement up of 48 relative to 47 indicates that the crown of 48 is buccal to the roots of 47. The apices of 48 have not altered in relation to the ID canal and are therefore in the same plane, immediately above the canal.

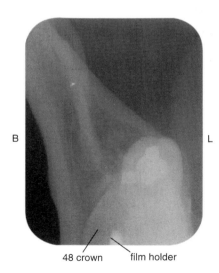

48 crown   film holder

Fig. 4.14c True occlusal projection using a periapical film packet confirms that the crown of 48 is buccal to 47, and the apices in the same plane as the roots of 47. The projection geometry involved directing the beam forwards from behind the angle of the mandible, projecting the image of 48 more

It is important to assess the radiograph using the highest point of observation first. An example in which this combination is useful is illustrated in Fig. 4.14.

Combinations that lend themselves to the BUILD assessment include:

- Panoramic and lower periapical, taken with an *upward* (negative) angulation.
- Upper oblique occlusal and panoramic.

4.5   USEFUL RADIOGRAPHIC COMBINATIONS

It has already been said that parallax can be applied to a combination of radiographs in which there is an inherent difference, and that difference is understood. There are a number of traditional combinations, and others that are less frequently considered. The following sections look at these in turn.

4.5.1   Periapicals

Two periapicals of essentially the same teeth need to have a horizontal difference incorporated in their execution if they are of the same type (i.e. if both paralleling technique, or if both bisecting angle technique). If one is paralleling and one bisecting angle then there will be an inherent vertical difference, except in the lower molar region where the vertical beam angulation will be very similar. Periapicals are of particular value when there is a need to separate roots when carrying out multiple canal endodontic treatment. Two conventional periapicals will provide images that are easiest to interpret (Fig. 4.12) and are easier to execute than attempting to incorporate specific angular differences.

The example shown in Fig. 4.15 is of a supernumerary tooth related to the root of 45. The two periapical films are centred on different teeth, so there is a horizontal difference in the tube position. To determine the position of the crown of the supernumerary relative to the root of 45 the apparent relationship must also be assessed horizontally. The crown appears to move in the same direction as the tube, and therefore it is relatively lingual. (In this same

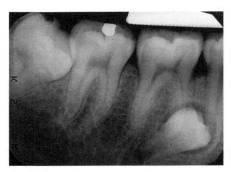

Fig. 4.15a The crown of the unerupted premolar is partially superimposed on the root of the last premolar evident in this radiograph: M 19.

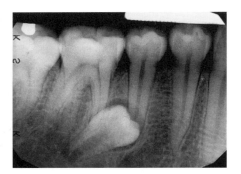

Fig. 4.15b The unerupted tooth is seen to be a supplemental premolar; both premolars are erupted. The X-ray tube has moved mesially and the mesial surface of the supplemental is now level with the mesial surface of the root of 45: it has moved in the same direction as the tube and is therefore lingual to 45.

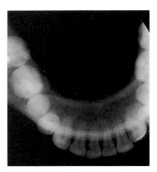

Fig. 4.15c True occlusal view taken at the same time gives a clear indication of the lingual position of the crown of the supplemental tooth, but provides no information about the 3-rooted 46

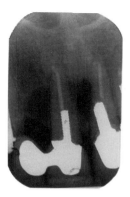

Fig. 4.16a The radiolucency mesial to the root of 21 is indicative of inflammatory change subsequent to a perforation during preparation for the post-crown. On this view taken with the X-ray tube centred over 11, the perforation is evidently mesial, but it may be to the facial or palatal aspect: F 79.

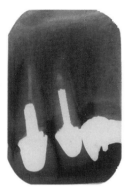

Fig. 4.16b The tube has been moved to the patient's left, centred over 22; the radiolucency and the end of the post have also moved to the left relative to the root, and are therefore palatal.

case the lower first molar has three roots which are only evident in one of the radiographs (Fig. 4.15b). Examination of the two taking into account the directional movement allows us to identify it as a disto-lingual root).

In endodontic treatment, and the subsequent restoration of the tooth, there is often a need for multiple views of a tooth. An unfortunate reason is when a lateral perforation occurs; accurate localization assists in deciding whether the situation can be resolved, and the direction of a surgical approach, if needed (Fig. 4.16).

4.5.2 Bitewings

A molar and a premolar bitewing of the same side differ in their centring point, and the images can then be examined for differences in a horizontal

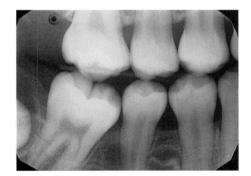

Fig. 4.17a On the bitewing radiograph the central ray is directed at 90° to the arch centred on 45; there is evidence of two developing supernumerary teeth positioned symmetrically between 44 and 45, and superimposed on the root of 45: M 15.

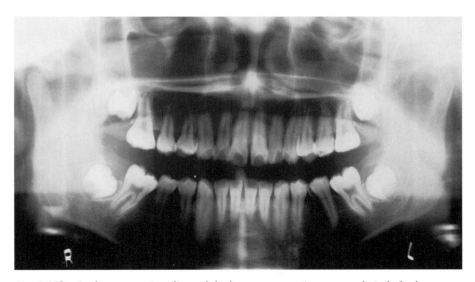

Fig. 4.17b In the panoramic radiograph both supernumeraries appear relatively further forward; the X-ray beam is passing through the teeth at an oblique angle, resulting in a more mesial observation point (similar to a more mesial bitewing).

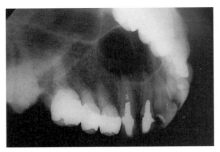

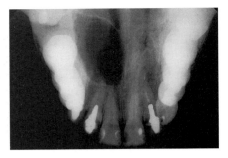

Fig. 4.18b   The oblique occlusal centred on the canine clearly shows the relationship between the lesion and the apex of 13, and the lack of involvement of the premolars. The mesial aspect of the lesion appears to involve the apex of 21, indicating that the cyst extends further buccally than the apex, as there was no involvement seen in the anterior occlusal.

Fig. 4.18a   An oval, radiolucent cystic lesion is associated with the roots of 11 and 12, and extends posteriorly into the palate: F 32.

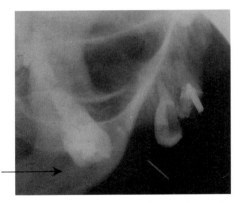

Fig. 4.19b   The tube has moved vertically to take the oblique occlusal, and the object has moved down, indicating its buccal position, in the cheek tissues. (Self-assessment: what anatomical feature is indicated by the arrow?)

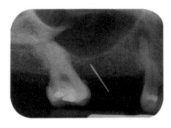

Fig. 4.19a   The slim, metal foreign body is superimposed on the alveolar ridge and mucosa on this paralleling periapical. It was not visible in the mouth, and the patient was unaware of its presence: F 44. Note the radiopaque calculus on mesial 17, the periapical area of radiolucency associated with the apex of 14, related to the gross caries, and the dilacerated root of 14.

direction. Superficially placed unerupted teeth in the region are likely to show up in bitewings, as well as on panoramic views, and it may be unnecessary to take additional views for the purpose of localization, provided there is a difference in the images in the two views. Figure 4.17 shows a case where two late developing supernumeraries are present in the lower right premolar region; the differences in the projected images of the erupted premolar teeth in the views available, allow the two views to be assessed as similar to two bitewings with different tube positions.

4.5.3   Occlusals

Oblique occlusals are essentially large bisected angle periapicals and can be used in an identical way, taking account of the effective difference in centring point in the horizontal direction (Fig. 4.18).

4.5.4   Combinations of different projections

Two different intra-orals

Any two intra-orals views which have been taken with a difference in their centring position, in either the horizontal direction or the vertical direction, may be used. Figure 4.19 illustrates the value of a paralleling periapical together with an oblique occlusal view where the difference in tube position is in the vertical direction; this can be assessed with SLOB, or BUILD if the occlusal is examined first.

Panoramic view combined with an intra-oral

Panoramic (or paralleling periapical) and maxillary oblique occlusal views provide good examples of such a combination. Figure 4.20 shows a panoramic radiograph and upper anterior oblique occlusal taken for the common problem of failure of eruption of an upper canine in a 14-year-old boy. Oblique occlusals may be taken of any region of the jaws; Fig. 4.21 illustrates the combination of a panoramic radiograph, and an oblique occlusal centred on the region of interest.

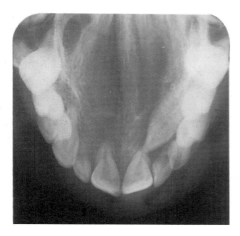

Fig. 4.20b A steep vertical angle has been used to take this occlusal radiograph; the crown tip of 23 is almost level with the apex of 21. The point of observation has moved up; the crown of 23 has also moved up and it is therefore palatal to 21.

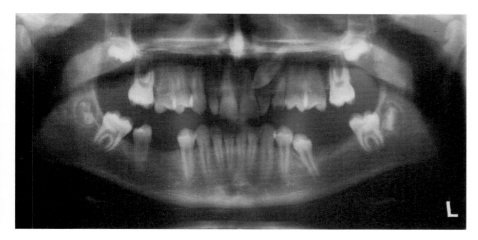

Fig. 4.20a 13 is erupted, 23 impacted, and 63 retained: the crown tip of 23 is half way up the length of 21 and there is obvious enlargement of the follicular space, indicative of dentigerous cyst formation: M 14. Note the peg-shaped upper lateral incisors; the root of 22 obscured by the more opaque mass of superimposed 23; 45 is in a very posterior position due to the early loss of 46 allowing it to drift distally as it erupts.

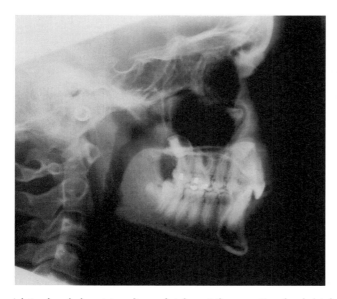

Fig. 4.21c A lateral cephalometric radiograph taken at the same time for skeletal assessment demonstrates the almost horizontal position of 13, and the relatively buccal position of the crown tip.

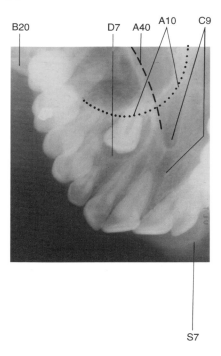

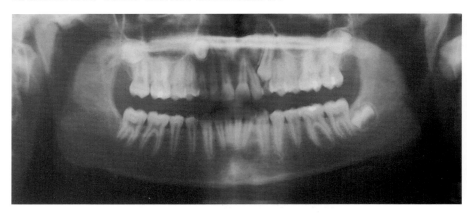

Fig. 4.21a   23 is in a normal alignment, although the region is crowded as depicted by the root displacement of 22; 13 is ectopically situated. It lies almost horizontally transverse to the arch with its full length higher than the apices of the nearby teeth. Careful examination of the image should enable detection of the palatal ridge, and that the buccal aspect of the tooth is superiorly placed. M 14.

Fig. 4.21b   The oblique occlusal is centred on 13 region and depicts the full length of the tooth. Examination, and application of the principles of parallax, determine that the crown tip is just buccal to the line of the arch (it has moved down to a lower level than the level of the apices of 12 and 14), and the root mass and apex are palatal. It is important to assess both ends of an object separately, in situations such as this where there is room for the reference plane to be crossed.

The presence of multiple views of a region may allow the decision to be checked, by assessing the images in both horizontal and vertical directions. The case illustrated in Fig. 4.22 is of a young boy with two upper midline supernumeraries, and divergence of the roots of the central incisors. In this situation the possibility exists for each end of each supernumerary to be in a different plane, and they must be assessed separately. The information obtained from the radiographs will influence the surgical approach as the

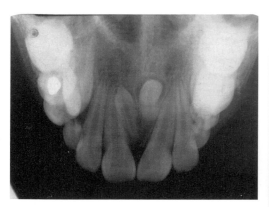

Fig. 4.22b   The X-ray tube has moved up for the occlusal: the right and left crown tips have moved up and down respectively, indicating their palatal and facial positions with respect to the central incisor apices. The apex of the SL has moved up, away from the root of the incisor and is palatal to it.

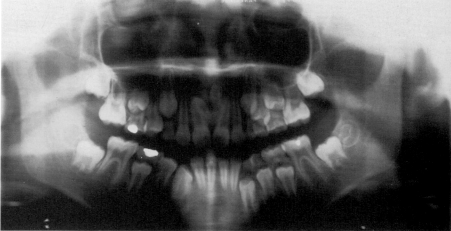

Fig. 4.22a   In addition to the unerupted canines and premolars there are two supernumeraries present in the upper midline region: both are inverted, the crown tip of the right one (SR) at a lower level than the apex of 11, and the crown tip of the left one (SL) at a higher level than the apex of 21: M 9.

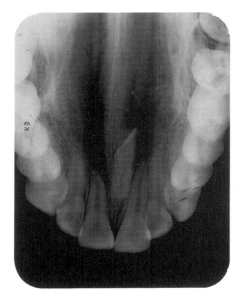

Fig. 4.23b The upper anterior occlusal view shows the full length of the tooth: the crown tip is much higher than the apices of 11 and 21 and is thereforepalatal to the incisors; the apex is much lower than the apices of 11 and 21 and is therefore buccal to the incisors, having moved in the opposite direction.

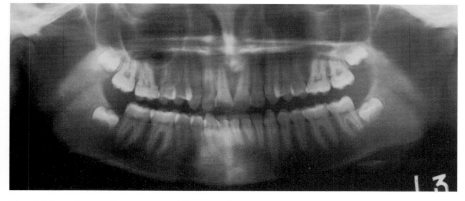

Fig. 4.23a A mesiodens is situated between the roots of 11 and 21, transverse to the arch and slightly lower than their apices: M 15 (see also Fig. 4.24).

crowns of all teeth, including supernumeraries, have a greater circumference than their roots.

4.6 POOR COMBINATIONS

The examples used throughout this chapter have generally utilized two different views, each providing a different image of the object to be localized, and altering its apparent relationship to other structures. Lack of thought when deciding on the views to be taken can result in two views which utilize such similar projection geometry that there is very little difference in the images.

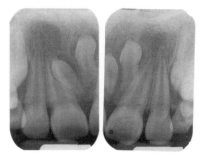

Fig. 4.22c Two paralleling periapicals were also taken, allowing horizontal assessment between each other. Although the root of 11 is only seen in one image it can be seen that the root of SR has moved in the same direction as the tube as its pulp canal is only clearly visible in the left periapical. The apex has however not moved. The apex of SL has moved in the same direction as the tube.

In summary, the position of the two supernumerary teeth with respect to the central incisors is:

SR (right) – crown tip palatal to root of 11
          – root palatal to root of 11 leading to a line of arch position of the apex
SL (left) – crown tip facial to root of 21
         – root and apex palatal to root of 21

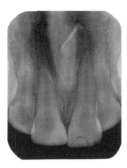

Fig. 4.23c A bisecting angle periapical was also taken at the same time (in 1985): the image and relations depicted are virtually identical to the upper anterior occlusal due to the similar geometry, and projection technique for these two views — only one of these images was required, and due to the known height of the supernumerary the occlusal is recommended.

LOCALIZATION USING DENTAL RADIOGRAPHY

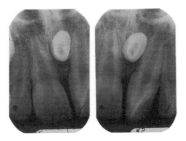

Fig. 4.24b Two paralleling periapicals taken to assist in localizing the precise position and orientation of the mesiodens; the images are very similar to each other and also to the panoramic radiograph as the projection geometry is virtually the same in all three views.

It is more useful to take bisecting angle intra-orals in conjunction with a panoramic radiograph in order to achieve a substantial difference in vertical angulation.

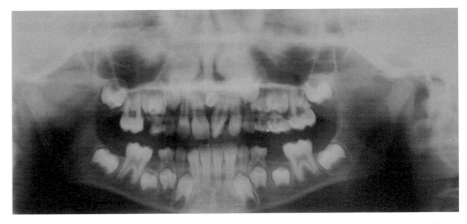

Fig. 4.24a A mesiodens is situated between the roots of 11 and 21, transverse to the arch and slightly lower than their apices. This is similar to the case depicted in Fig. 4.23, except that there is a closer relationship in this example between the mesiodens and 21; the incisor is rotated through 90°, bucco-mesially: M 9.

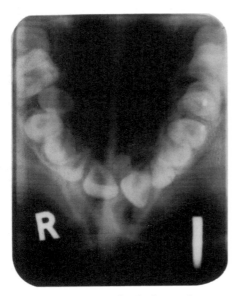

Fig. 4.24c A vertex occlusal taken at the same time as the other films shows the mesiodens crossing the arch with its crown palatal; it is difficult to see the image of the mesiodens due to the nature of the overlying structures and an upper anterior oblique occlusal would have provided a clearer image which would have been more straightforward to interpret.

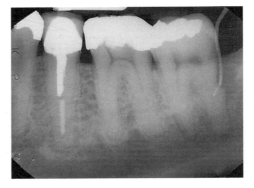

Fig. 4.25 Gutta percha (GP) point within a periodontal pocket, illustrating the depth of the pocket; clinically, it was known to extend on to the buccal aspect of the tooth: M 45.

Figures 4.23 and 4.24 illustrate this problem, and the captions indicate which views are superfluous, and suggest the most appropriate combinations in each case.

4.7 RADIOPAQUE MARKERS

Inclusion of a known object such as a gutta percha (GP) point is helpful in visualizing the extent of periodontal pockets and discharging sinuses (Figs 4.25 and 4.26). Another application of this principle is the use of metal inclusions in an acrylic base plate in order to accurately locate retained roots which are not closely related to any useful features. The same base plate can then be used during the surgical procedure to assist in accessing the root at the correct place, thus avoiding unnecessary bone removal.

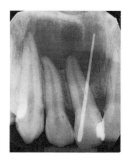

Fig. 4.26a Gutta percha (GP) point placed in a chronic sinus opening to determine the source of infection; 11 is implicated as the cause of the extensive bone destruction: M 20

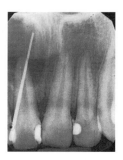

Fig. 4.26b The change in relation of the GP point with the root of 21 demonstrates the buccal position of the sinus.

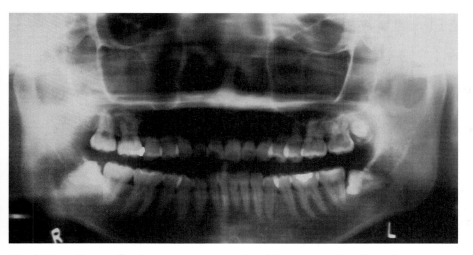

Fig. 4.27a Two small radiopaque masses were detected on panoramic radiography; asymptomatic, it was decided to determine how they were related to the left parotid duct: F 21.

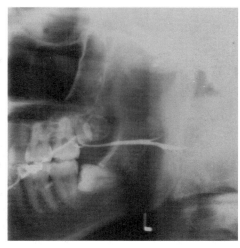

Fig. 4.27b Radiopaque contrast in the left parotid duct clearly demonstrates that there is no connection between the two. The differential diagnosis for the radiopacities includes phleboliths and lymph node calcification.

It is occasionally necessary to employ the use of non-solid contrast agents, as illustrated by the case in Fig. 4.27 in which sialography was used as an investigative tool.

4.8   SELF-ASSESSMENT EXAMPLES

The examples in Figs 4.28–4.34 can be used to practise applying the principles of localization outlined in this chapter. In each case the reader should consider what the effective difference is, in the X-ray tube position, between the views provided. Examine the images looking at how the object of interest moves in relation to a chosen reference in that same direction. There are additional questions to be answered in some of the examples; the answers are provided in the next section. The previous examples can also be used for self-assessment for revision purposes.

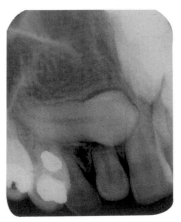 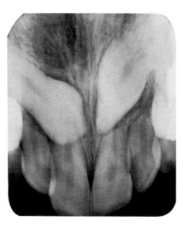 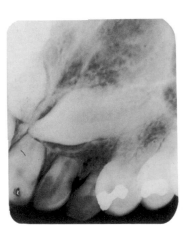

Fig. 4.28   What is the relationship of the impacted canines with the incisor teeth? F 18.

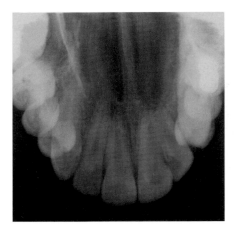

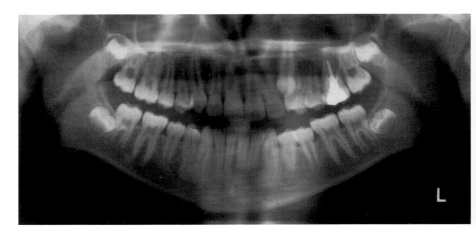

Fig. 4.29   The upper left canine is impacted, and should be palpable. From the radiographs what is its relationship to the arch? M 11.

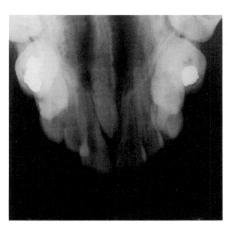

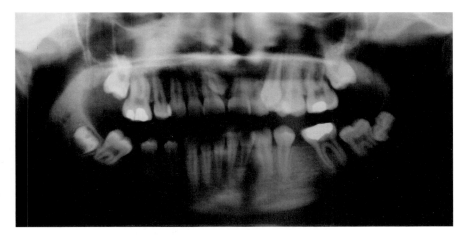

Fig. 4.30 A supernumerary tooth is evident in close association with 11. What is the relationship, and how is 23 related to the arch? M 12.

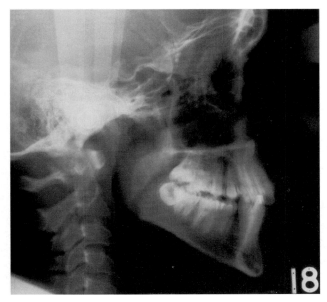

Fig. 4.31b The lateral cephalometric view clearly demonstrates the buccal inclination of the tooth coronally.

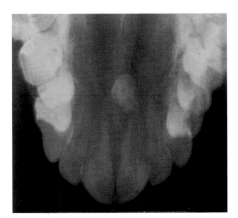

Fig. 4.31a How is the supernumerary tooth related to the upper left central incisoir? M14.

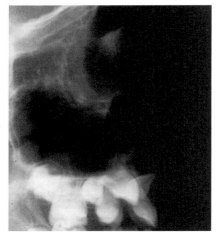

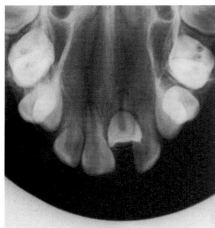

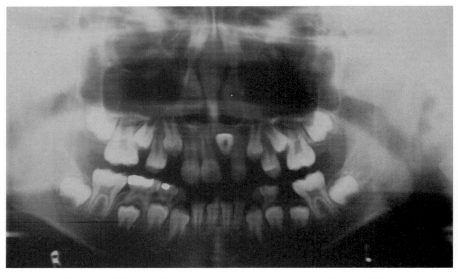

Fig. 4.32   The upper left central incisor is unerupted, and shows evidence of dilaceration. What is the alignment of the root and crown, and how is the tooth related to the arch? F 8.

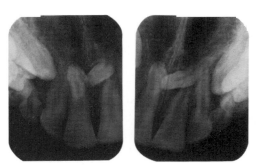

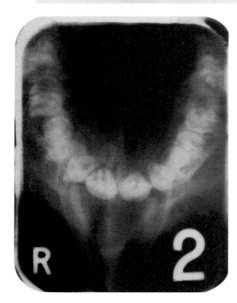

Fig. 4.33b   Vertex occlusal taken at the same time (in 1985) clearly demonstrates the right supernumerary: the left supernumerary is not well demonstrated due to its partial superimposition on the images of 21, 22, and 23.

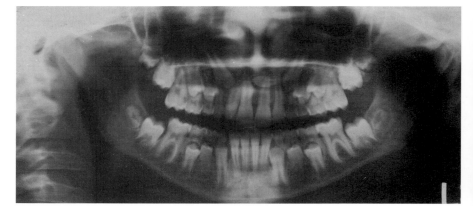

Fig. 4.33a   How many supernumerary teeth are present? What is the relationship of the impacted supernumerary and canine teeth to the erupted teeth? M 9.

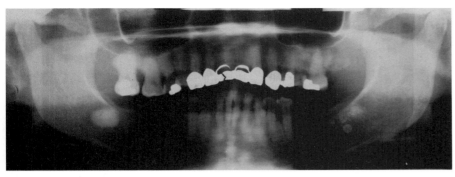

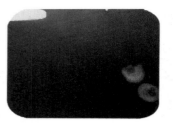

Fig. 4.34b A film placed between the cheek and the teeth confirms the presence of two of the opacities within the cheek; they were also palpable.

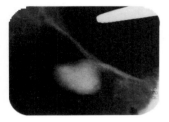

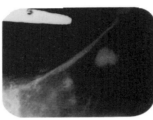

Fig. 4.34a Where are the radiopacities which appear to be in the lower molar regions on the panoramic view? What do you think they might be?

4.9   ANSWERS TO SELF-ASSESSMENT EXAMPLES

Fig. 4.19   The arrowed structure is the zygoma

Fig. 4.28   The three periapical views demonstrate impacted canines and root resorption of 12, 21, and 22; the crowns of 13 and 23 must therefore be in the same plane as these roots. The root of 11 is in a different plane as there is no resorption: horizontal parallax indicates that the crown of 13 is palatal to the root of 11. The normal alignment of incisors is such that the root of the upper lateral tends to be more palatal than the central.

Fig. 4.29   23 is relatively superficial with its crown tip level with the alveolar crest/enamel margin of 24 in the panoramic view. In the upper anterior oblique occlusal view the crown tip of 23 has moved down to be level with the buccal cusp of 24 indicating its relatively buccal position.

Fig. 4.30   In the panoramic radiograph the supernumerary is super-imposed on 11 and partially between 11 and 21; its apex is lower than the apex of 11; the tip of the crown of 23 is midway up the crown of 22. In the upper anterior occlusal view, the apex of the supernumerary has moved to above the apex of 11 and is therefore palatal; the crown tip of this tuberculate supernumerary is at the same level as in the panoramic view and is therefore in the line of the arch — a surgical approach from the palatal aspect would be advocated; the crown tip of 23 has moved down and is therefore buccal.

Fig. 4.31   In the panoramic radiograph an inverted mesiodens is present with its apex superimposed on the apex of 21; the crown is much broader than the apex which suggests that it may be more palatal. In the upper ante-rior occlusal view the apex of the mesiodens has moved up to just above the apex of 21, and the length of the tooth has become shorter indicating that the crown tip is buccal relative to its own apex — the supposition based on the horizontal dimensions of the supernumerary in the panoramic film was incorrect, indicating the risk of relying on size and distortion effects when interpreting panoramic images.

Fig. 4.32   The dilacerated 21 is related to trauma during development. The panoramic, oblique occlusal, and lateral projections are almost at right angles to each other and enable accurate localization of each part of the tooth with respect to the rest of the tooth and other structures. The root is almost horizontal across the arch: it is seen full length in the occlusal view and in cross-section in the panoramic view. The crown is directed supero-buccally; the incisal edge is very superficial and should be palpable: F 8. (See also Fig. 6.8.)

Fig. 4.33   There is a horizontal supernumerary seen in the panoramic view overlying the roots of 21 and 22 with its crown mesial and crossing the midline. The two bisecting angle periapical views clearly show two supernumeraries; careful further examination of the panoramic view demonstrates an increased opacity over part of the root of 11, which corresponds to the position of the tooth on the right. The three films provide a horizontal tube shift between the two periapicals and a vertical tube shift between the panoramic and periapical views. The following positions can be determined: the supernumerary on the right is palatal to the root of 11 and inverted; the supernumerary on the left has its crown in the line of the arch and its apex palatal to the arch; there is a mild degree of dilaceration between the crown and the root.

Fig. 4.34   The single radiopacity on the right is within the mandible as its position has not altered in the two views. The degree of radiopacity is similar to sclerotic bone, or a root mass (from 48). On the left-hand side there are four radiopacities, exhibiting two different degrees of opacity: in the bisecting angle periapical, taken with an upward directed beam, two are unchanged in position, and are of a similar nature to the mass on the right; the other two have moved up and are clearly within soft tissue, buccal to the mandible. These two are less radiopaque, almost circular, with a suggestion of layering in their appearance. Their appearance is consistent with a diagnosis of phleboliths.

The need to localize structures in relation to each other is referred to elsewhere in this book, where further examples can be found. Localization, using dental radiography, is not an exercise to be carried out for its own sake, but should be seen as an important component of the complete examination, providing information that helps to build-up the knowledge required about the patient.

5   Coronal and pericoronal changes

5.1   INTRODUCTION   94
5.2   NORMAL APPEARANCE AND DEVELOPMENTAL CHANGES   94
5.3   ABNORMALITIES   95
    5.3.1   Abnormal development   **95**
    5.3.2   Trauma   **104**
    5.3.3   Inflammatory   **104**
    5.3.4   Cystic   **104**
    5.3.5   Metabolic   **104**
    5.3.6   Iatrogenic   **106**
    5.3.7   Artefact   **106**

5 Coronal and pericoronal changes

5.1 INTRODUCTION

The crown of a tooth is the only anatomical part normally accessible to the examining clinician. The outer surface can be seen using direct vision with the exception of the proximal portions in contact with other teeth. A number of other methods of examination can also be utilized.

The following methods of examining the crowns of erupted teeth are used:

- Visual
  — direct vision
  — assisted vision: FOTI (fibre-optic trans-illumination)
- Tactile
  — dental probe, or other instruments
- X-rays
  — radiographic

X-rays enable visualization of the subsurface structures, and the surface areas not otherwise accessible. They should, however, only be utilized as a diagnostic tool when the other available methods are inadequate, either for reasons of access or sensitivity.

5.2 NORMAL APPEARANCE AND DEVELOPMENTAL CHANGES

The following tissues and structures are included in this region:

- Enamel
- Dentine
- Pulp
- Cementum
- Periodontal ligament
- Dental socket
- Alveolar bone
- Gingiva
- Dental crypt
- Dental follicle
- Dental papilla

The appearance of certain features can be influenced by a number of points which should be borne in mind:

1. Soft tissue structures are only shown due to their delineation by adjacent hard tissue structures or air.
2. Cementum is not distinguishable from dentine on radiographs.
3. There is a natural variation of appearance of any tissue form even within a single image, caused by the quantity in the path of the X-ray beam (Fig. 5.1), and the nature of the adjacent structure.

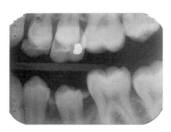

Fig. 5.1 Left bitewing radiograph of late mixed dentition; the opacity of the crowns of 24 and 25 is increased by the remaining shells of 64 and 65; the deciduous enamel is much thinner than that on the permanent teeth: M 13.

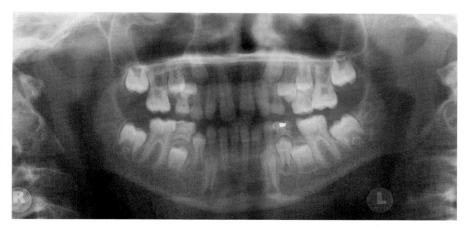

Fig. 5.2 Early mineralization of 38 and 48: M 10.

Prior to mineralization the developing tooth germ is detected as a circular or oval radiolucency (see Figs 3.27 and 4.17), well demarcated from the surrounding alveolar bone. The first sign of mineralization occurs at the enamel–dentine junction, beneath the cusps in canines, premolar, and molar teeth (Fig. 5.2), and beneath the incisive edges in the incisors. The crowns of unerupted teeth are surrounded by a follicle (the reduced enamel epithelium), seen radiologically as the follicular space between the enamel and the surrounding bone. As the tooth erupts, the reduced enamel epithelium merges with the oral epithelium and disappears.

5.3   ABNORMALITIES

5.3.1   Abnormal development

The teeth may develop abnormally, or acquire an abnormal appearance as a result of external factors. Many of the developmental anomalies affect the crown of the tooth and these are listed below and illustrated in Figs 5.3–5.12. In addition to these examples those abnormalities more particularly affecting the root structure are illustrated in Chapter 6.

Form

Reduced size
Increased size
Double teeth
Altered morphology:
    Invaginations/evaginations
Additional dental structures:
    Supplemental and supernumerary teeth
    Odontomes
    — compound
    — complex
    — dilated (invaginated)
Hypoplasia/hypomineralization:
    Single tooth (Turner tooth)
    Multiple teeth
Amelogenesis imperfecta
Odontodysplasia

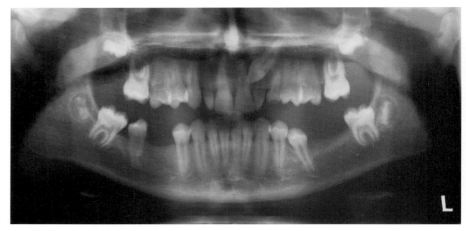

(a)

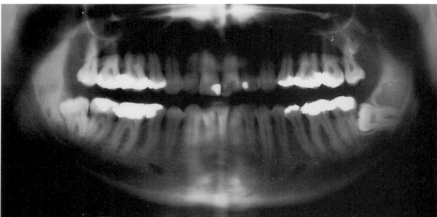

Fig. 5.3

(a) Reduced crown size of upper lateral incisors, commonly referred to as peg-shaped incisors; the follicle associated with 23 is enlarged but within normal limits: M 10.

(b) Denticle in 28 position; all other third molars are of normal size: M 26.

(b)

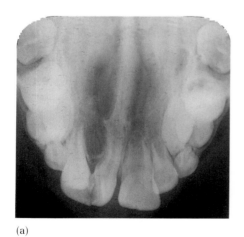

(a)

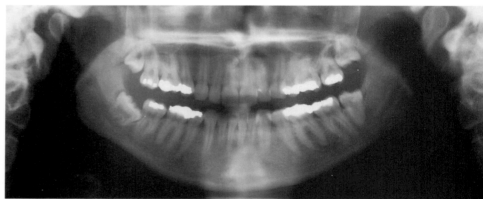

(b)

Fig. 5.4

(a) Increased size of 21, root and crown; 12 and 22 are present and normal; 11 has fused coronally with a supernumerary, or gemination has occurred — the roots are separate.

(b) Increased size of 48 (note also upper supernumerary): F 22.

(c) Fusion of 51 and 52; the permanent successors are not affected: F 3.

(d) Fusion of lower incisors and upper third molar; extracted teeth.

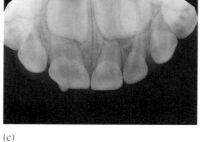

(c)

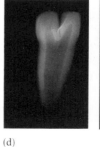 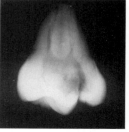

(d)

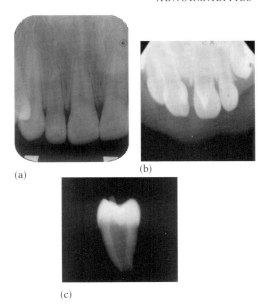

Fig. 5.5
(a) Invagination of enamel of 12; enamel caries
12 m, 11 d, 21 m; dentine caries 11 m: F 16.
(b) Evagination or talon cusp of 51 and 61: M 1.
(c) Evagination in extracted Leung's premolar.

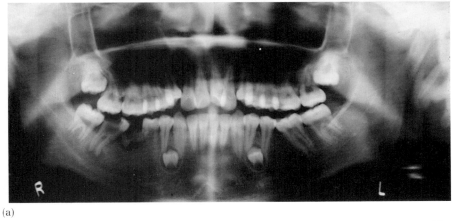

Fig. 5.6
(a) Late-developing supplemental lower premolars:
F 17.
(b) Multiple supernumerary teeth: F 19.

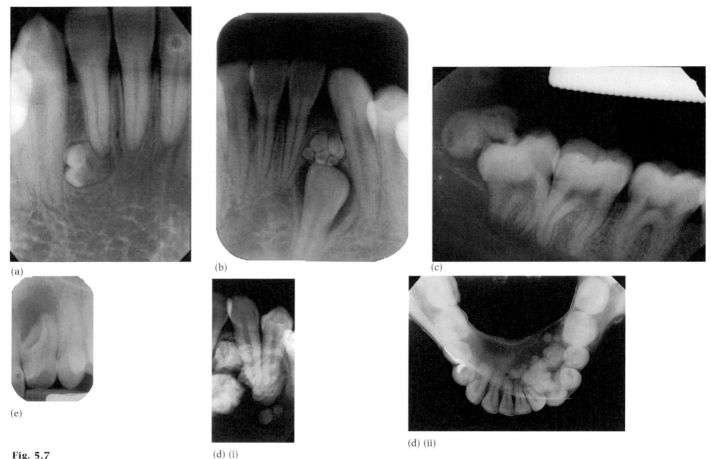

Fig. 5.7

(a) Denticle between 42 and 43: M 18. (b) Compound odontome preventing eruption of 32: F 15. (c) Complex odontome related to DA 48: F 17.
(d) (i and ii) Extensive compound odontome formation, with dentigerous cyst formation: F 22. (e) Dilated odontome formed by geminated, invaginated 22: F 16.

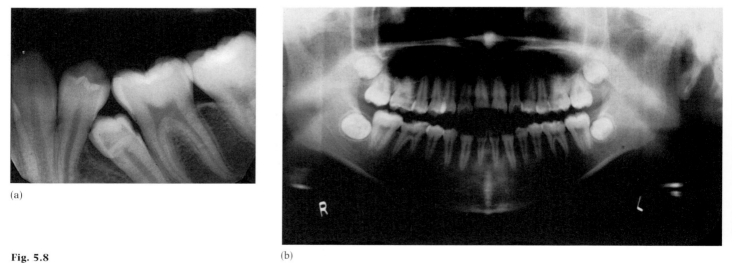

Fig. 5.8

(a) Hypoplastic 35 (Turner tooth) caused by periapical infection associated with 75: M 13. (b) Chronological hypoplasia affecting all incisors, canines, and first molars; congenital absence of 23, 32, and 42: F 14.

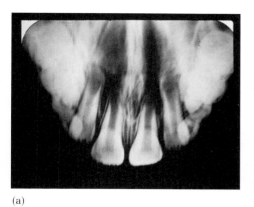

(a)

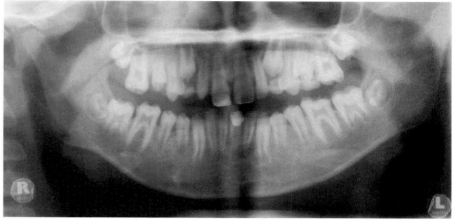

(b)

Fig. 5.9
(a) Amelogenesis imperfecta causing notching of incisal edges. (b) Amelogenesis imperfecta resulting in generalized thin, poor-quality enamel: M 11.

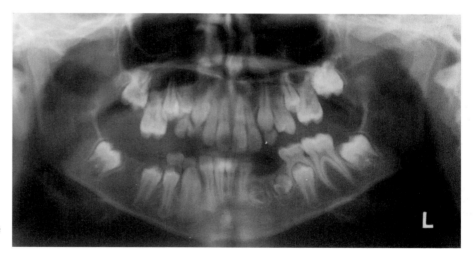

Fig. 5.10 Regional odontodysplasia affecting the lower left canine/premolar segment: M 9.

Position

Transposition
Submerging
Transmigration
Ectopic

The various development anomalies show a tendency to affect particular teeth; the lateral incisor, second premolar, and third molar are more frequently affected than other teeth, due to their development as the last in each series of tooth type (see also Chapter 3). A number of the anomalies are self-explanatory but the following notes are provided to clarify some of the conditions.

Form

Double teeth. This occurs when two tooth germs fuse together, or a single tooth germ partially divides (gemination): the appearance may be identical in the two situations. Increased size of teeth is likely to be an expression of this phenomenon.

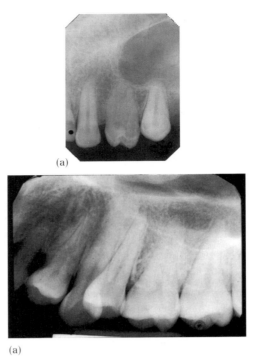

(a)

(a)

Fig. 5.11
(a) Transposition of 23 and 24; 24 is rotated bucco-distally.
(b) Transposition of 23 and 24: F 25.

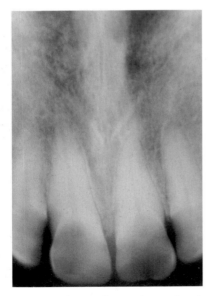

Fig. 5.13   Loss of coronal tissue due to chronic chemical erosion: M 27.

Invaginations and evaginations. It is not uncommon to find palatal invagination of enamel in the upper lateral incisor (Fig. 5.5a): also known as dens in dente (a tooth within a tooth), the condition predisposes to early loss of vitality if caries occurs in the invagination. Rarely, the condition is also seen in central incisors.

Evaginations involve an additional coronal extension of pulp tissue covered by a 'cusp' of dentine and enamel. This occurs in two situations: in incisor teeth, permanent and deciduous, as a cusp to one side of the palatal surface — referred to as a talon cusp due to its eccentric position (Fig. 5.5b); in premolar teeth, as a central cusp arising from the mid-occlusal position. Premolars are predominantly affected in persons of Mongoloid races, and were first described in Singapore: they are often known as Leung's premolars (Fig. 5.5c). These extra cusps are prone to traumatic injury, acute (causing fracture), or chronic occlusal trauma resulting in secondary dentine formation: both situations can result in early loss of vitality.

Supplemental and supernumerary teeth (Fig. 5.6) have been referred to in Chapter 3 (p. 55), and are most frequently seen in relation to the upper midline, and sites close to the lateral incisor, second premolar, and third molar.

Odontomes are developmental abnormalities of the combined dental tissues, with three main expressions:

1. *Compound*: multiple denticles present within a single follicle; each denticle has a crown and root, the dental tissues having a normal relationship to each other (Figs 5.7a and b)

2. *Complex*: a single mass in which the dental tissues do not have the normal relationship to each other (Fig. 5.7c)

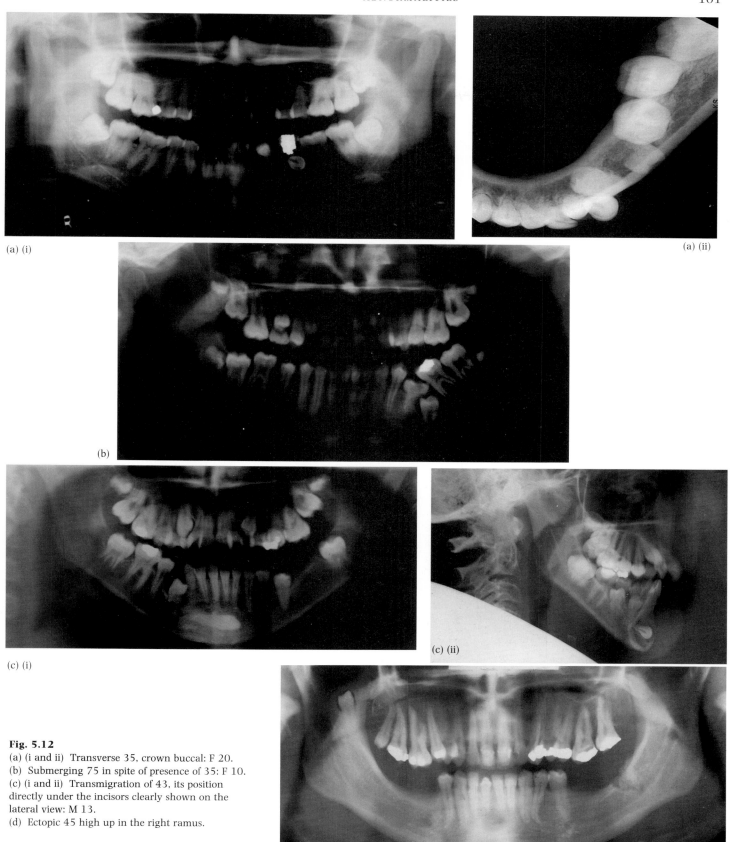

(a) (i)

(a) (ii)

(b)

(c) (i)

(c) (ii)

(d)

Fig. 5.12
(a) (i and ii) Transverse 35, crown buccal: F 20.
(b) Submerging 75 in spite of presence of 35: F 10.
(c) (i and ii) Transmigration of 43, its position
directly under the incisors clearly shown on the
lateral view: M 13.
(d) Ectopic 45 high up in the right ramus.

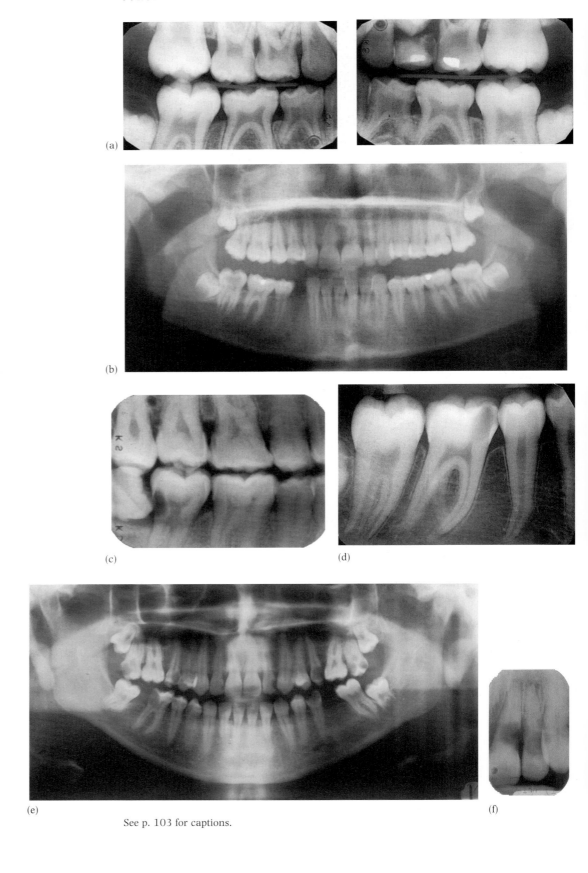

See p. 103 for captions.

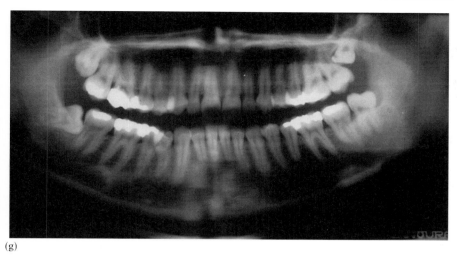

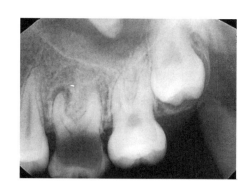

(h)

(g)

Fig. 5.14

(a) Proximal surface caries in deciduous teeth: 55m, 54m, 64d, 65m, 75m, 74d, and enamel caries in 85m and d: M 7. (b) Deep caries 47occ.; proximal caries 14m, 24m, 25m and d, 26d, 36m, 46m: F 14. (c) Low-level proximal caries in 47d, related to MA partially erupted 48: M 50. (d) Isolated deep caries 46 m; note the three roots: M 13. (e) Widespread advanced caries, with cavitation. (f) Root caries due to exposed root surface associated with periodontal disease: M 61. (g) Caries in unerupted 28m: F 35. (h) Cavitation in 26 associated with the common sequel of periapical inflammatory bone resorption: F 24

3.   *Dilated (invaginated)*: the extreme form of an invaginated tooth, there is usually gross malformation and these teeth have a poor prognosis (Fig. 5.7e)

Hypoplasia and hypomineralization. External influences on developing teeth can result in an interruption of normal formation, expressed as altered form or degree of mineralization. Single teeth that are not infrequently affected are premolars, due to their close proximity to the roots of the deciduous molars; the affected tooth is often referred to as a Turner tooth (Fig. 5.8a). Multiple teeth are affected when there is a severe systemic upset, resulting in bands of hypoplasia at different levels according to the precise stage of development each tooth type had reached. In the example (Fig. 5.8b), the upper lateral incisors are not affected as they had not commenced mineralization at the critical time, whereas the central incisors, canines, and first molars are all affected; this can be determined to have occurred during the first few months of life, and is hence referred to as chronological hypoplasia.

Amelogenesis imperfecta is manifested as either a defect in the enamel matrix or a defect in enamel mineralization, which is most striking radiologically (Fig. 5.9). These conditions are inherited and affect all the teeth.

Regional odontodysplasia affects all the dental tissues, in a specific group of teeth, in which the teeth do not form properly (Fig. 5.10).

Position

There are many expressions of abnormal position of teeth, ranging from the abnormalities seen daily due to crowding, to the ectopic tooth that has migrated to a site remote from its normal position (Fig. 5.12d). Transposition involves two teeth that erupt into each other's position, and most frequently involves the canine due to the late timing of its eruption (Fig. 5.11). Teeth that fail to maintain their correct position in the occlusal plane are referred to as submerging, the commonest expression of this is the retained deciduous molar with no permanent successor. In Fig. 5.12b the permanent successor is present, the deciduous tooth has extensive caries, and 46 has tilted mesially, which may have influenced the situation. Transmigration is where a tooth migrates and crosses the midline; it is most frequently seen in connection with mandibular canines (Fig. 5.12c).

5.3.2 Trauma

The radiological appearance and resultant changes, attributable to physical trauma, are covered in Chapter 10. The enamel, and subsequently dentine, can also be damaged by repeated chemical attack, particularly from acidic liquids such as stomach regurgitation, citric fruit juices, and many proprietary soft drinks. The widespread loss of tissue (Fig. 5.13) has a quite different appearance to the tooth loss associated with caries or physical trauma.

5.3.3 Inflammatory

● Caries
● Internal resorption

Caries is manifested radiologically as a radiolucency affecting the hard tissues of the teeth. It commences at the surface, but remineralization, due to fluoride supplements, can result in an intact surface with subsurface destruction. A variety of carious lesions are depicted in Figs 5.5a and 5.14.

Occasionally internal resorption is seen in teeth for no apparent reason; it will only be evident clinically at a late stage, when the crown may be so weakened as to be unsaveable.

5.3.4 Cystic

The follicle of the tooth and the periodontal ligament both incorporate epithelial tissues, and can undergo cystic change if the appropriate circumstances arise. The dentigerous cyst classically incorporates the crown of the tooth from which it arises (Fig. 5.15), and occurs in relation to permanent teeth. The eruption cyst (Fig. 5.16) is similar to the dentigerous cyst but, as its name implies, is associated with erupting teeth and is either naturally transient, the tooth erupting through it, or is surgically marsupialized. Both these cysts envelop the crown. Cystic lesions clearly related to the crown, but not fully enclosing it suggest a differential diagnosis of odontogenic keratocyst or paradental cyst.

The paradental cyst (Fig. 5.17) is classically related to a partially erupted tooth, and pericoronitis has been implicated as an aetiological factor. Unlike the dentigerous cyst, which arises from the reduced enamel epithelium, the paradental cyst arises from epithelial cell rests and histologically resembles the radicular cyst.

5.3.5 Metabolic

Once formed, the enamel cannot alter in structural terms, except for the demineralization changes caused by caries and other forms of acid attack, and remineralization aided by fluoride. The systemic metabolism can however have a profound effect on the developing tissues, and the structure and content of the hard tissues can be influenced at this stage. There will only be

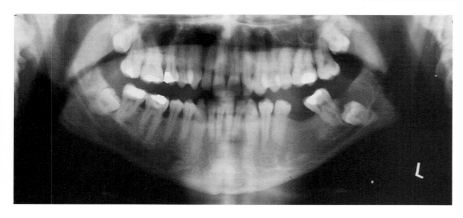

Fig. 5.15 Dentigerous cyst arising from follicle of 38: M 28.

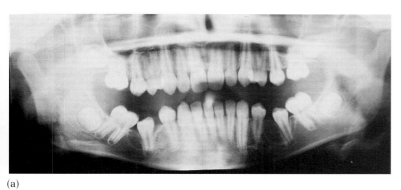

(a)

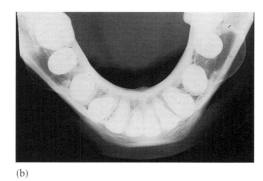

(b)

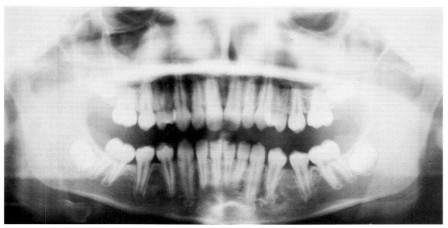

(c)

Fig. 5.16
(a and b) Eruption cysts associated with 35 and 45: M 13.
(c) 6 months later with no treatment the teeth are erupting normally.

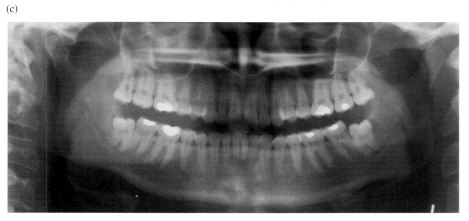

Fig. 5.17 Paradental cyst associated with partially erupted 38: F 22.

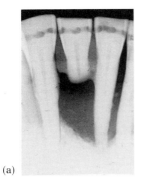

(a)

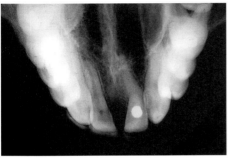

(b)

Fig. 5.18
(a) Preparation for splinting in advanced periodontal disease: F 45.
(b) Veneers on canines and lateral incisors to mimic lateral and central incisors, centrals lost due to trauma; note the sclerosed pulp in 22 which shows mild dilaceration: M 15.

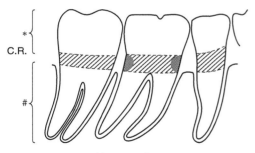

*   crown covered by enamel

\#   roots surrounded by alveolar bone

C.R. cervical radiolucency where reduced attenuation of beam

≫ ≪   in the mesial and distal margins there is even less tooth material, and darker areas soometimes appear, mimicking cervical caries

Fig. 5.19   Diagrammatic representation of cervical radiolucency affecting a molar tooth, manifested as either a band of radiolucency, or mesial and distal radiolucencies mimicking cervical caries.

radiologically evident changes when there is a substantial physical change in the nature of the tissues, as occurs in chronological hypoplasia (Fig. 5.8b).

5.3.6   Iatrogenic

Tooth preparation, for the purpose of placement of restorations, should be recognizable by the outline form (Fig. 5.18); problems can arise, however, when there is no restoration present, a radiolucent restoration, or the cavity shape simulates a carious cavity.

5.3.7   Artefact

Cervical radiolucency is a not uncommon artefact that frequently mimics cervical caries. The name is derived from the location and appearance, although there are two common appearances (Fig. 5.19 and 5.20; see also Fig. 7.23). Both are predominantly seen in relation to the posterior teeth, and are variations of the same effect. The cervical region of the tooth presents a lesser amount of hard tissue to the X-ray beam, when transmitted in a bucco-lingual direction (bitewings, periapicals, and panoramic images), than the enamel-covered crown and the bone-encased roots. Even when there is no loss of height of the alveolar bone, there is a narrow band in this cervical region of the tooth where this is always the case. The X-ray beam is attenuated less as it passes through this region; if the difference in attenuation is sufficient then a radiolucent band will result. In addition, the oval cross-section of the premolar and molar teeth results in an even more reduced attenuation mesially and distally.

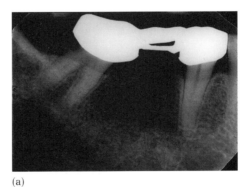

(a)

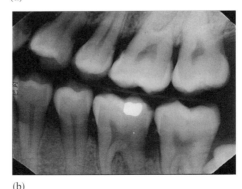

(b)

Fig. 5.20
(a) Band appearance of cervical radiolucency crossing 45 and 47; co-incident cervical caries in 47d: F 60.
(b) Cervical radiolucency accentuated by calculus on 35 and 36: M 30.

6 Pulp and root changes

6.1 INTRODUCTION   108
6.2 NORMAL STRUCTURE AND DEVELOPMENT   108
6.3 ABNORMALITIES   110
    6.3.1 Abnormal development   **110**
    6.3.2 Trauma   **114**
    6.3.3 Inflammatory   **115**
    6.3.4 Metabolic   **115**
    6.3.5 Idiopathic   **116**
    6.3.6 Iatrogenic   **116**
    6.3.7 Secondary to other pathology   **116**
6.4 SHORT ROOTS   116

6   Pulp and root changes

6.1   INTRODUCTION

The pulp and mineralized tissues of the root are intimately related to each other in normal development, and their response to adverse influences. This chapter will illustrate the range of abnormalities that can affect the component tissues, and their variation from the normal appearance.

6.2   NORMAL STRUCTURE AND DEVELOPMENT

The tissues that constitute the pulp and root of the tooth are all connective tissues, the living pulp consisting of blood vessels, neural tissue, loose connective tissue, and odontoblasts. The pulp develops from the dental papilla and at all stages of its formation, and when fully formed, is radiolucent on radiographs. The shape of the pulp chamber and root canals define the outline of the pulp. A non-vital pulp and an empty pulp chamber also appear radiolucent and there is no discernible difference in their interaction with the X-ray beam. Decisions about the state of vitality of a pulp can only conclusively be made with sophisticated tests that indicate blood flow; the presence of a functioning neural component can be tested with a variety of pulp testing tools including electrical and thermal stimulation.

Radiological features may however be *indicative* of the state of vitality of the pulp, for example, presence of a carious lesion in continuity with the pulp chamber is highly indicative of a non-vital or irreversibly damaged pulp, and the presence of a root filling fully obliterating the pulp chamber and canals is clear evidence that the tooth must be non-vital. In contrast to this, an area of periapical radiolucency, although frequently suggestive of underlying pulpal changes, is not conclusive evidence of a non-vital tooth as there are other pathological lesions that may present in this way in relation to vital teeth (Fig. 7.27).

The root of the tooth consists of dentine and cementum. Radiologically, these tissues are indistinguishable due to their similar levels of mineralization and effective atomic numbers. Figure 6.1 illustrates the characteristic radiological appearance of the various stages of root development in two children. Note, particularly, the following appearances:

(1)   early root formation, and the division into multiple roots;
(2)   the continuity of the image of the space occupied by the tooth follicle around the full circumference of the developing tooth with the forming pulpal tissues (dental papilla);
(3)   immediately prior to the apical constriction forming
(4)   the completed apex.

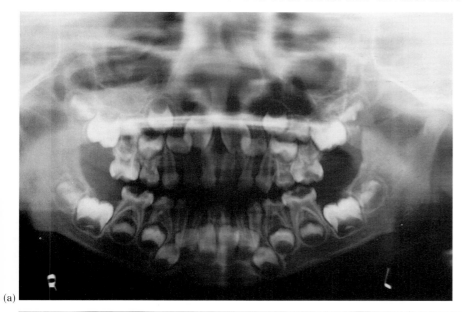

(a)

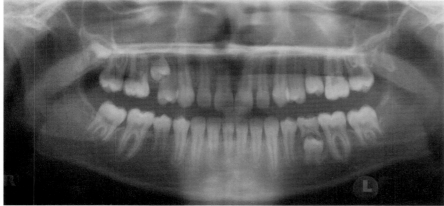

(b)

Fig. 6.1
(a) Age 4 years 6 months: the incisors and first molars have commenced root development.
(b) Age 11: the root length of 37 is increasing; the apex of 34 is about to form; the apex of 44 has just been completed.

At all stages prior to formation of the apex the advancing front of the root forms an acute angle, and outlines the flaring shape of the forming pulp canal. This shape gives rise to the term 'open apex', which is a normal finding in any tooth that is still actively developing. In a tooth that should have completed its development it is a sign that the pulp became non-vital during development.

Figure 6.2 illustrates the opposite end of the scale, when extensive narrowing of the pulp canal has resulted from deposition of secondary dentine. This is a normal physiological process, although increased formation of secondary dentine also occurs as a pathological response to abnormal stimuli, and in many teeth the quantity of secondary dentine will be influenced by both mechanisms. Radiologically, there is no discernible difference between physiological and pathological secondary dentine. At the same time as there has been continued hard tissue formation on the inner walls of the pulp, there is frequently a continuing addition to the cementum covering of the tooth so that the external morphology may also undergo a gradual change.

A knowledge of some key dates in the chronology of tooth development is helpful in deciding whether the appearance of a particular tooth is normal for the age of the patient or not. In this respect, most texts on dental anatomy

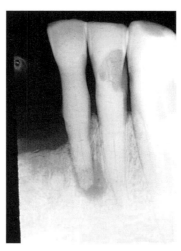

Fig. 6.2 In the elderly, the formation of secondary dentine, and further deposition of cementum alter the root appearance: M 74.

include information that is based on studies using Caucasian populations; other groups may exhibit variations in timing, and there are also variations according to the different sexes.

6.3 ABNORMALITIES

6.3.1 Abnormal development

There are a number of abnormalities which affect the root tissue and structure, ranging from those considered to be variations of normal, due to their frequency, to clear abnormalities.

The following abnormalities will be illustrated:

- altered root number
- altered root morphology
- dysplastic conditions

Root number

Each member of both the deciduous and permanent dentition has a usual number of roots; any variation to this can be considered an abnormality, although in some population groups the variation may be so common, as to be anticipated as the normal. As the root mass is divided into an increasing number of roots, each one becomes thinner and less easy to detect. They will also be less easy to instrument in endodontic treatment, and more prone to fracture during extraction. Three-rooted lower molars are not uncommonly seen (Fig. 6.3); in addition to altered number, the lower molar pulpal morphology can exhibit a C-shape in cross-section, although it appears normal radiologically. The two-rooted upper first premolar is generally accepted; this is less common in lower premolars and three roots are very unusual (Fig. 6.4). Even more unusual are two-rooted canines (Fig. 6.5). Multiple canals are, however, seen even in incisors (Fig. 6.6).

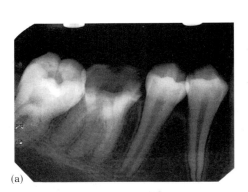

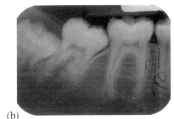

Fig. 6.3
(a) Grossly carious 3-rooted 46: M 15.
(b) 4-rooted 47: F 15.

Root morphology

There is a wide range of 'normal' root morphology, particularly the variations seen in third molars. Variations considered outside the range of normal include dilaceration, taurodontism, and fusion/gemination of teeth.

Where there is a particularly marked bend in the root this is referred to as 'dilacerated', and can cause problems with eruption.

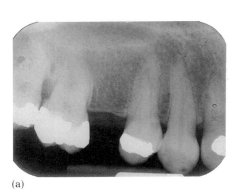

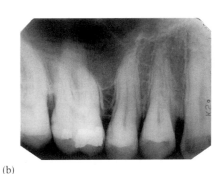

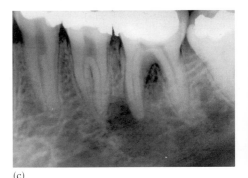

(a)   (b)   (c)

Fig. 6.4
(a) Normal 2-rooted 14. (b) 3-rooted 14: M 25. (c) 2-rooted 35, exhibiting taurodontism.

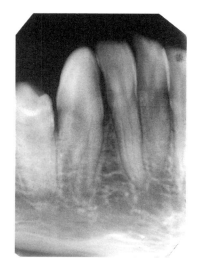

Fig. 6.5   2-rooted 43: M 12.

Dilaceration

di = twice, two, double.
lacerate = mangle or tear.

The term is used to refer to any sharp bend in a tooth normally, but not exclusively, affecting the root portion (Figs 6.7 and 6.8). The dilaceration may be parallel to the plane of the film, when it can be seen on a single radiograph, or at an angle to the plane of the film, requiring localization views to be taken.

Taurodontism

The name of this trait is derived from the word *taurus*, Latin for *bull*, and *dont*, meaning *tooth*: thus, bull-like tooth. It only occurs in teeth with two or more roots, and is manifested by an increase in height of the coronal pulp chamber, and relatively short separate roots: the overall height of the tooth is unaltered. There is a wide range of appearances of taurodont teeth; all have in common the altered ratio of pulp chamber to full pulp length (Figs 6.4c and 6.9). In multi-rooted teeth the normal ratio of the height of the pulp chamber to the full length of the pulpal structure is 1:5. When this ratio is 1:4 or greater, that is the pulp chamber is at least a quarter of the full length of the pulp, then the tooth can be described as taurodont. This condition most frequently affects the molar teeth.

Enamel pearls (Fig. 6.9) are occasionally seen at the furcation of multi-rooted teeth.

Double teeth (Fig. 6.10) can occur as a result of fusion of two tooth germs, or gemination (twinning) of a tooth germ. Fusion can involve normal series teeth and supernumerary teeth (see also Chapter 5). Double teeth can also exhibit invagination of the enamel into the pulp chamber, sometimes to the point of formation of a dilated odontome (Fig. 6.11).

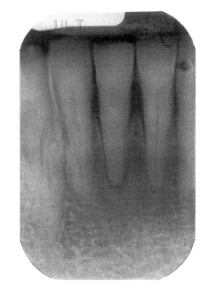

Fig. 6.6   Two canals in 42.

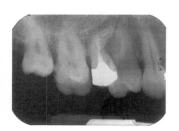

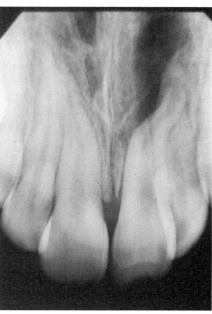

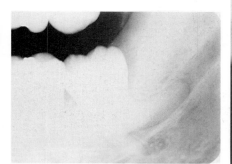

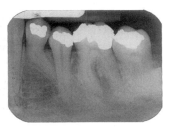

Fig. 6.7   Dilacerated roots of 15, 21, 34, and 38 in different patients, where eruption has still occurred

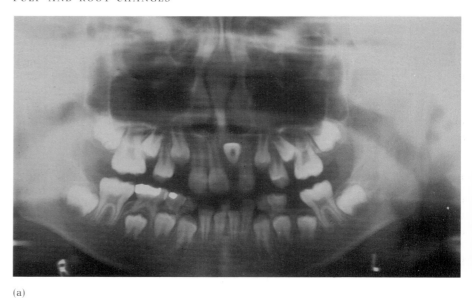

(a)

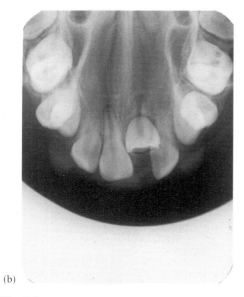

(b)

Fig. 6.8
(a) Dilacerated 21, preventing eruption.
(b) The different direction of movement of the incisal
edge and root apex enable their relative positions to
the arch to be determined*: F 8.

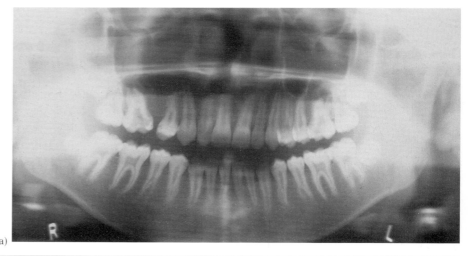

(a)

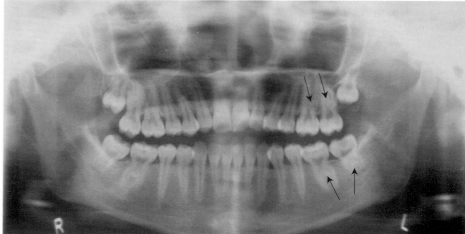

(b)

Fig. 6.9   (a) Taurodont lower premolars: M 14.
(b) Taurodont molar teeth and enamel pearls
(arrowed): F 20.

Concrescence

The roots of two teeth may be fused by cementum, most frequently involving the upper third molar tooth. It is critical to consider this possibility when intending to extract either the upper second or third molar, if their radiographic images demonstrate an intimate relationship. The word's derivatives mean *to grow together*, and this situation may be an early or late developmental change. It is not necessarily possible to determine radiographically if teeth are joined, or merely in close proximity.

Premature arrest of development

Cessation of development prior to natural completion of the root tissues occurs as a result of two main reasons: (1) irreversible interruption of the blood supply to the tooth; and (2) irreversible inflammatory change in the pulpal tissues. Examples of these different causes of a similar radiological finding will be found in Chapter 10 on dental trauma. The most reliable sign of arrested development is the presence of an open apex in a tooth which should have completed development according to the age of the patient (Fig. 6.22a), combined with a short root length.

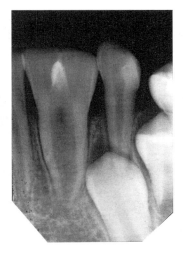

Fig. 6.10 Double tooth in 32 position; there is an additional lingual tubercle at the junction of the coronal portions: M 10.

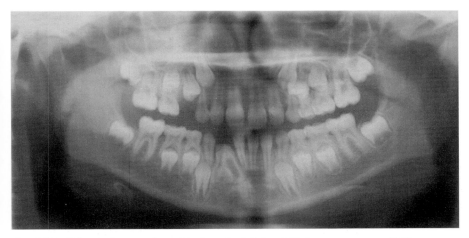

Fig. 6.11 Dilated odontome formed by invaginated, fused 42 + supernumerary: F 18.

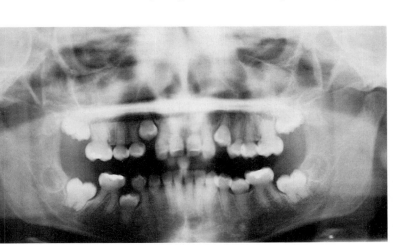

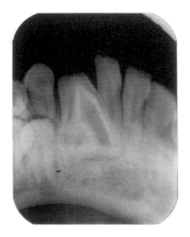

Fig. 6.12 Dentinogenesis imperfecta.

Dysplastic conditions

Dentinogenesis imperfecta and dentine dysplasia
There are recognized classifications of developmental disorders that affect the microscopic and macroscopic structure of the various dental tissues. Of special importance when considering the pulp and root are the developmental disorders primarily affecting dentine structure and formation. In dentinogenesis imperfecta there is a tendency for teeth to have bulbous crowns, and early obliteration of the pulp canals (Fig. 6.12). In dentine dysplasia, the teeth exhibit short roots, obliteration of pulp canals, and multiple periapical areas of radiolucency (Fig. 6.13).

Odontodysplasia
This condition affects the whole structure of the tooth, and normally affects a segment of adjacent teeth. The teeth are referred to as ghost teeth, and they exhibit abnormalities of all component tissues (Fig. 6.14); there is an associated tendency to delayed eruption, or complete failure to erupt.

6.3.2 Trauma

Trauma to the dentition can have a profound effect on the hard and soft tissues of the teeth. The causes of dental trauma, and the associated radiological appearances are covered in Chapter 10.

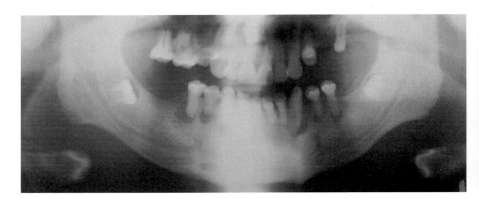

Fig. 6.13 Dentine dysplasia: M 20

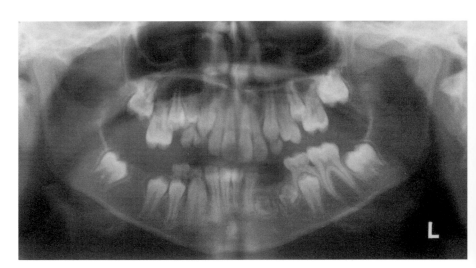

Fig. 6.14 Regional odontodysplasia affecting the lower left canine/premolar segment: M 9.

6.3.3. Inflammatory

The pulp is normally protected from changes in the oral environment by the protective covering of enamel surrounding the crown. Damage to the enamel causes the dentine to become the first line of defence, and immediately opens up a communication channel to the pulp through the dentinal tubules. The dimensions of a tubule lumen will naturally decrease during a tooth's lifetime as peritubular dentine is laid down, but in the younger tooth little protection will be afforded by the dentine. The vital pulp has the ability to lay down secondary dentine, as a physiological age change, and in response to irritation, both resulting in a reduction in size of the pulp chamber and canals (Fig. 6.15).

Pulp stones are a variation of secondary dentine. They are frequently found in teeth throughout both jaws, and are demonstrable by their relative radiopacity (Fig. 6.16); more common in posterior teeth, they can occur in anterior teeth. They exist in continuity with the inner walls of the pulp chamber or as free entities; the two types may be indistinguishable radiologically. Their presence will influence the ease of conducting endodontic treatment.

Irreversible inflammatory change of the pulp can result from a number of causes, ranging from caries to chronic occlusal trauma; regardless of the cause the ultimate changes will be the same, and will lead on to periapical inflammatory conditions (see Chapter 7).

Internal resorption is an expression of pulpal inflammation sometimes associated with traumatized teeth, or occurring for no known cause (Fig. 6.17); for the resorption to occur the pulp must still be vital.

External resorption (Fig. 6.18) by contrast is caused by osteoclastic activity, and affects both vital and non-vital teeth. It is a not infrequent complication of re-implanted teeth, where its occurrence is closely linked to the status of the pulp; endodontic treatment often results in cessation of the resorption.

6.3.4   Metabolic

Hypercementosis is linked to Paget's disease of bone, as well as being a feature associated with increasing age (Fig. 6.19).

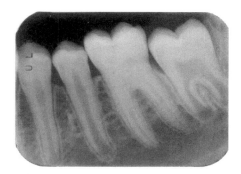

Fig. 6.15   Idiopathic secondary dentine formation in 36: F 12.

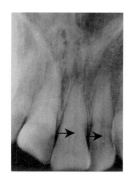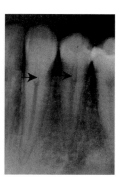

Fig. 6.16   Pulp stones (arrowed) in anterior and posterior teeth: F 18.

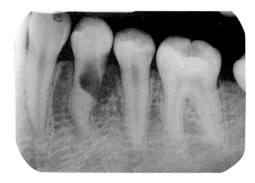

Fig. 6.17   Internal resorption in 34: F 17.

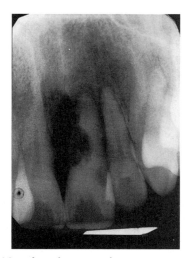

Fig. 6.18   Idiopathic external resorption in 21: M 59.

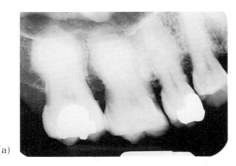

(a)

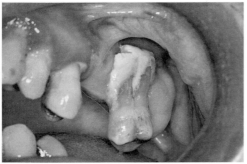

(b) (ii)

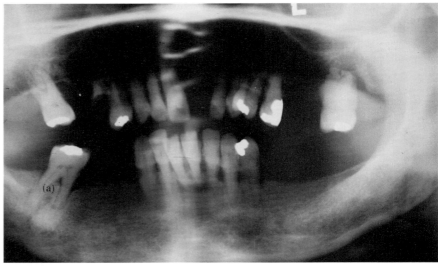

(b) (i)

Fig. 6.19
(a) Hypercementosis affecting 17 and 16: F 57.
(b) 27 appears to have hypercementosis (i), the appearance being caused by excessive deposits of calculus (ii).

6.3.5   Idiopathic

Altered appearance of root tissues is not always attributable to a known cause; the case illustrated in Fig. 6.15 is a good example of a case where there was no known reason for the extensive production of secondary dentine in this vital tooth.

6.3.6   Iatrogenic

The iatrogenic changes that predominantly affect the pulp and root tissues are usually related to endodontic treatment and apicectomy, and are readily recognizable in relation to their appearance and the patient's treatment history.

6.3.7   Secondary to other pathology

Any pathological process intimately related to the root of a tooth can affect it, causing resorption or displacement. There are numerous examples throughout the text which illustrate the changes that can be seen.

6.4   SHORT ROOTS

The term 'short root' is purely descriptive, and does not in itself indicate the cause for this relatively common appearance. There is an extensive list of causes, ranging from the normal to the illusionary, caused by radiographic technique. They have been grouped together here for illustrative purposes;

many are associated with non-vital teeth, and these are also illustrated in Chapter 7.

Causes of radiological 'short roots'

- Normal developing *, and fully formed deciduous roots ^
- Normal resorbing deciduous #
- Normal but short ^
- Arrested development *
- Resorbing, pathological #
    with or without bone replacement
        bone normal or sclerotic
    (for a fuller account of this phenomenon see Chapter 7)
- Exfoliation ^
- Trauma
- Iatrogenic
- Radiographic ^

The symbols ^, #, and * have been used to denote a characteristic radiological appearance of the apex, which is useful in establishing a differential diagnosis, and in particular to rule out possible causes:

^ the apical end has a completely normal 'bullet-shaped' appearance, and other factors need to be taken into account in order to determine the cause of the short root (Figs 6.20a,c; 6.21a,b; 6.24c);

the apical end of the root is blunt and the pulp canal is slim with near parallel sides; the appearance indicates that the root has previously been fully formed (Figs 6.20b; 6.23a,b; 6.24a,b).

* the apical end of the root has an 'open apex' appearance, the walls of the root flaring outwards to finish with an acute angle between the outer and inner root margins (Figs 6.22a,b);

Examples of some typical appearances of short roots are demonstrated in Figs 6.20–6.25. Further relevant examples can be found in other chapters.

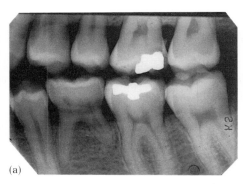
(a)

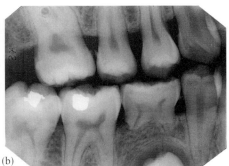
(b)

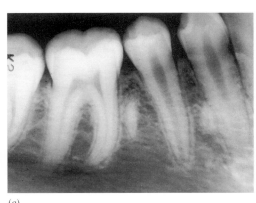
(c)

Fig. 6.20
(a) Normal fully formed deciduous roots of 75; the tooth is still present with no permanent successor: M 32.
(b) Resorbed deciduous roots of 85; 45 is present but has ceased active eruption and new bone has been laid down: F 20.
(c) Retained fragments of 85 surrounded by healthy bone: M 12.

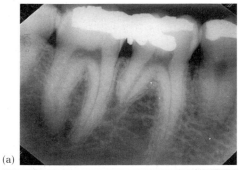

(a)

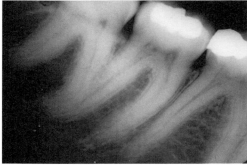

(c)

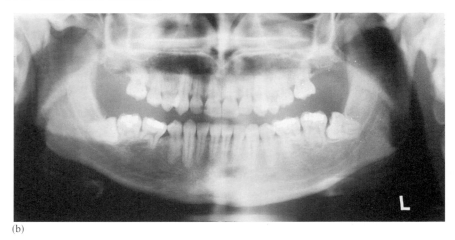

(b)

Fig. 6.21
(a) Short, normally shaped distal root of 46; no history of orthodontic treatment; ? normal variation: M 21.
(b) Short normally shaped roots of lower first and second molars: F 23.
Where all roots of a tooth are abnormally short, the tooth is at risk if periodontal disease occurs.
(c) Contrasting long roots of lower molars: M 31.

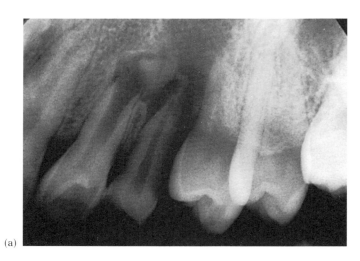

(a)

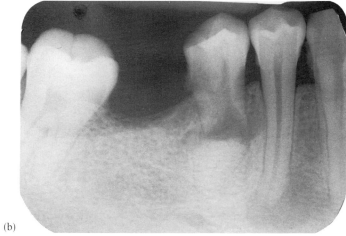

(b)

Fig. 6.22
(a) Arrested development of invaginated 22: M 17. (See also Fig. 3.32.)
(b) Arrested development of coronal portion of 45; the dental papilla must have been traumatically separated, and has continued to form a normal apical portion of the root: M 35.

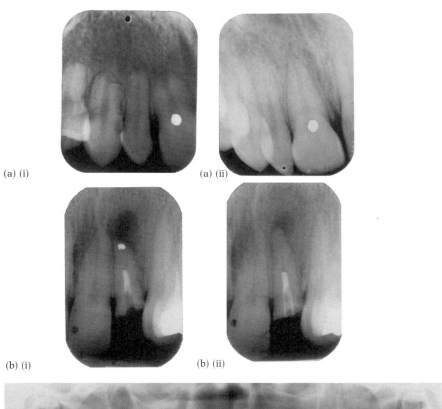

(a) (i)   (a) (ii)

(b) (i)   (b) (ii)

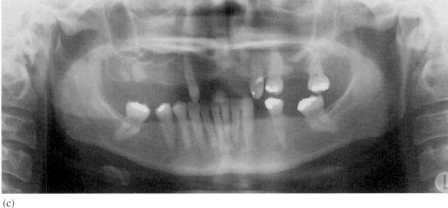

(c)

Fig. 6.24
(a) Resorption of root of 12 due to orthodontic tooth movement (i), compared to pre-treatment film (ii).
(b) Short root resulting from apicectomy of 22 (i), compared to pre-treatment film (ii).
(c) Displaced palatal root of 26, during extraction: F 49.

*Fig. 6.8: The incisal edge is buccal to the arch, the root apex is palatal (See also Fig. 4.32.)

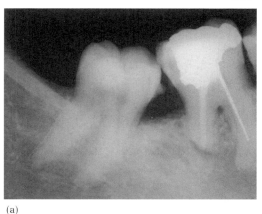

(a)

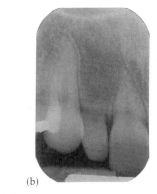

(b)

Fig. 6.23
(a) Resorbing distal root of 46 with normal bone replacement: M 34.
(b) Resorbed root of 12 due to path of eruption of 13; complete replacement by normal bone: F 20.

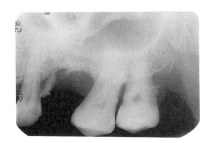

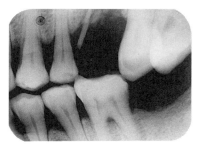

Fig. 6.25 Radiographic shortening of retained root fragment of 26, caused by change in vertical beam angulation: M 61.

7 Bone: periapical and periodontal

7.1   INTRODUCTION   122
7.2   NORMAL PERIODONTAL AND PERIAPICAL STRUCTURES   122
       7.2.1   Anatomical radiolucencies   **123**
       7.2.2   Anatomical radiopacities   **125**
7.3   INFLAMMATORY CHANGES   126
       7.3.1   Periapical   **126**
       7.3.2   Periodontal   **132**
7.4   NON-INFLAMMATORY PATHOLOGICAL PERIAPICAL
       CHANGES   133

7 Bone: periapical and periodontal

7.1 INTRODUCTION

The use of radiographs to assist in the diagnosis of periodontal and periapical disease must always be supplementary to a thorough clinical examination. Accurate interpretation of the radiological findings requires information about the status of the teeth that is not available from the radiographic images.

An understanding of the normal appearance, and variations of anatomical features closely related to the teeth, is needed to provide a sound basis for interpreting potential abnormalities. The section on normal structures includes detail about a number of features which can give rise to confusion, when they occasionally mimic pathological lesions.

The inflammatory changes which result in radiological changes of the dental supporting structures are reviewed in the sections on periapical and periodontal inflammatory change. There is often considerable overlap of these two regions, and changes that affect both are included in the section in which they have the greatest relevance.

7.2 NORMAL PERIODONTAL AND PERIAPICAL STRUCTURES

Erupted teeth are supported in the alveolar bone by the fibres of the periodontal ligament, which originate from the root cementum, and insert into the Sharpey fibre bone of the tooth socket, and into the cervical gingiva. The hard tissue components of the periodontium are well demonstrated in radiographic images, but the soft tissue components are only seen by virtue of their interface with hard tissues or air (see Chapter 2).

Within the jaws and teeth there are a number of anatomical features that appear on radiographs as radiolucencies, or radiopacities. This provides the potential for confusion to arise, particularly with regard to the radiolucencies:

(a) if any such feature is superimposed on a part of a tooth, most particularly the apex; and

(b) when a patient's symptoms indicate that something is probably wrong, but no clear explanation can be isolated.

The presence of such a radiolucency in these situations may encourage the clinician to abandon further investigation. Three straightforward tests are useful, however, to assist in making the correct decision as to whether the image in question represents a normal or abnormal feature:

1. A positive sensitivity test can rule out periapical pathology secondary to loss of pulp vitality.

2. Identification of normal anatomical features related to the root of the tooth (e.g. an intact lamina dura, or even a clear periodontal ligament

space around the apex of a tooth). Visualization of these features ensures a high probability that the *periapical radiolucency* is not an inflammatory lesion arising from the tooth.

3. In the event that the first two suggestions are inconclusive then radiographic localization techniques can be applied (Chapter 4) in order to determine whether the feature is separate from the apex.

An example of a situation in which the wrong diagnosis can be suggested is shown in Fig. 7.1: the tooth is non-vital and has been root treated, adding support to the idea of a pathological lesion. Careful examination of both radiographs demonstrates the normal periapical structures; the radiolucent area changes position in the two radiographs.

7.2.1   Anatomical radiolucencies

The anatomical radiolucencies with a potential for superimposition on the apex of a tooth can be classified according to the type of feature they represent. They are listed below, and are incorporated in the lists and illustrations of anatomical features in Chapter 2. Figure 7.2 illustrates a variety of features exhibiting close proximity to the apices of teeth.

Foramina
These are round or oval in cross-section. They are only clearly demonstrable on radiographs if the X-ray beam passes through them at, or nearly at, 90° to the surface of the bone in which they are situated. When the X-ray beam passes though at an oblique angle there is too much superimposition of normal bone to result in a clear image of the foramen. Because of their shape, superimposition of a foramen over the apex of a tooth is the commonest feature that mimics a 'periapical radiolucency'.

The following foramina present in the jaws have the potential to be radiographically superimposed on a tooth apex:

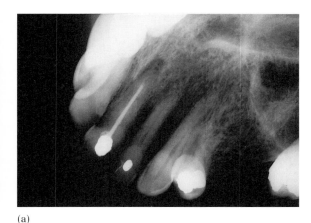

(a)
Fig. 7.1
(a) Periapical radiolucency clearly associated with 21: F 69.
(b) The radiolucency is now situated between the roots of 11 and 21, and is caused by the incisive foramen.

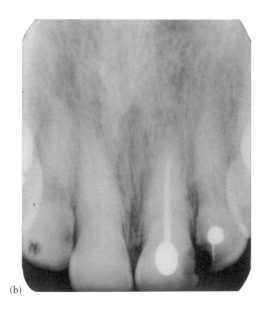

(b)

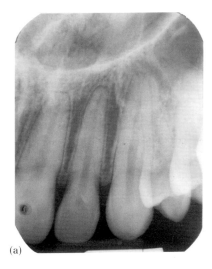

(a)

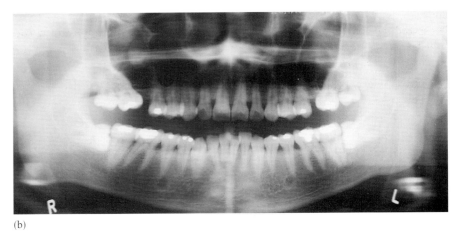

(b)

periapical area

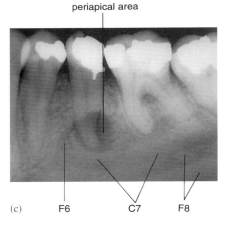

(c)   F6   C7   F8

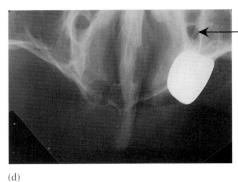

(d)

Fig. 7.2
(a) Anterior extension of maxillary sinus superimposed on apices of 23 and 24.
(b) Mental foramen at apex of 45: M 17.
(c) Mental foramen adjacent to true periapical area of bone resorption, related to pinned amalgam restoration in 35: F 32.
(d) Left lacrimal duct related to palatal apex of 26; there is also a residual radicular cyst in the right maxilla: F 63.

— mental foramen
— lingual foramen
— incisive (nasopalatine) foramen
— greater palatine foramen

Air cavities
All cavities containing air are relatively radiolucent compared to the immediately adjacent structure. Portions of these cavities may be radiographically superimposed on apices:

— oral cavity
— maxillary sinus
— nasal cavity

Neurovascular and other canals
Visualization of a considerable section of a canal should not present a problem with accurate identification, but short sections included near the edge of a radiographic image frequently mimic pathology:

— inferior dental (alveolar) canal
— superior alveolar vessel grooves
— miscellaneous nutrient canals
— lacrimal duct

Bone depressions

These reduce the thickness of cancellous bone between the opposing cortical plates, and result in a much sparser, or apparently indistinguishable, trabecular pattern. The two areas most likely to cause this problem are:

— the incisive fossa in the maxilla
— the submandibular fossa

Bone trabecular pattern

The appearance of the trabecular pattern of cancellous bone is subject to considerable variation between individuals, and also as a result of physiological and pathological influences throughout the course of an individual's life. Visualization of a large region as in a panoramic radiograph usually presents no problem in relation to 'periapical radiolucencies'. However, when only a small area is shown, or the viewer is mentally geared up to detecting pathological change, then considerable confusion can result from a sparse trabecular pattern. Figure 7.3 is an example of a periapical radiolucency related to the apices of a lower third molar. The tooth is partially erupted, but has no evidence of coronal pathology; this should alert to the likelihood that there is no pathology. In such a situation, if the tooth is to be removed, the opportunity should be taken to examine the bone directly, at least visually, provided the inferior dental canal and neurovascular bundle are not put at risk.

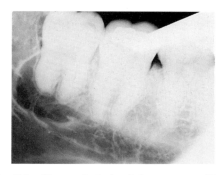

Fig. 7.3 Clear periapical radiolucency caused by trabecular pattern, and the inferior dental canal; the lamina dura is evident: F 21.

7.2.2 Anatomical radiopacities

The features which cause a local increase in opacity of the bone are usually more extensive than their radiolucent counterparts, and therefore less likely to cause confusion (Fig. 7.4). It is worth noting them, however:

Processes
— the zygomatic process and zygoma
— mylohyoid ridge
Bone margins
— the outline of the maxillary sinus
Tori
— mandibular
— palatal

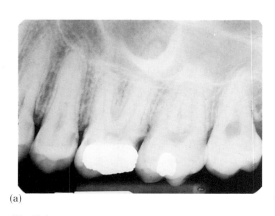

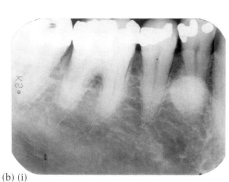

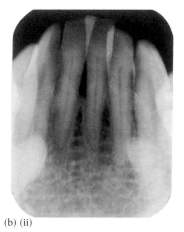

(a) (b) (i) (b) (ii)

Fig. 7.4

(a) The zygomatic process crossing the distopalatal root of the 4-rooted 26.(b) (i) Mandibular torus superimposed on apex of 44: M 53. (b) (ii) The tube shift has caused the opacity to move mesially, proving its relatively lingual position; the condition is symmetrical.

7.3   INFLAMMATORY CHANGES: PERIAPICAL AND PERIODONTAL

7.3.1   Periapical

> *Periapical*
>
> *peri* = round, about.
> *apex* = tip, top, pointed end;
>   plural: apexes/apices.

Periapical inflammatory changes will affect the periodontal ligament, and can affect the cortical bone of the tooth socket, the root of the tooth, and the alveolar bone extending from the tooth.

The inflammatory response that initiates the changes which will be evident on radiographs, are sequelae of a variety of situations, the commonest of which is pulpal death. Various situations may be implicated and can be classified as follows:

External influences, including:
— abnormally erupting teeth
— adjacent pathology, benign and malignant
Abnormal occlusal forces
Inflammatory origin including:
— irreversible pulpal pathology
— severe periodontal disease

Loss of vitality

Loss of pulpal vitality can be directly attributable to caries or trauma, and influenced by underlying factors. The various factors can be considered under the following categories, and are illustrated in Chapters 5, 6, and 10:

Developmental (predisposing to other direct factors)
— dens invaginatus
— dens evaginatus
Inflammatory
— caries
— periodontal lesions (perio-endo lesions)
Trauma, acute
— fracture
— loss of apical blood supply
— iatrogenic (cavity preparation/polishing)
Trauma, chronic
— attrition
— abrasion
— occlusal forces
— erosion
— iatrogenic

Abnormal occlusal forces can arise from an irregular dentition, altered masticatory or other occlusal habits, or iatrogenically from restorations, or following orthodontic treatment. Excessive pressure on single teeth may cause inflammation in the periodontium. The periodontium is a closed system bounded by the hard tissues of the tooth and its socket. As a result, the only

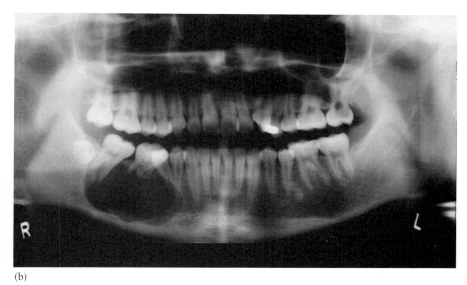

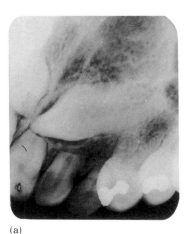

(b)   (a)

Fig. 7.5   Root resorption caused by:
(a) 23 erupting in the same plane as the roots of 21 and 22:F 18. (See also Fig. 4.28.) (b) Cystic ameloblastoma causing resorption of apices of 46: M 15. (See also Fig. 8.21.)

potential for adapting to the increased tissue fluid that is generated in an inflammatory situation is for the tooth to become slightly extruded, and radiographically this results in an apparent widening of the periodontal ligament space. Clinically, such a tooth usually exhibits tenderness to occlusally applied forces, and is commonly referred to as TTP (tender to percussion).

Other external influences exerting pressure on the root, can cause resorption of normal structures (Fig. 7.5). Recognition of the existence of an ectopic tooth, or underlying pathology, assists in determining the cause of the problem; treatment of the underlying cause should result in the resorption being halted.

The majority of teeth that have associated periapical inflammatory change fall into the group related to pulpal or periodontal problems. The inflammatory response of the periapical tissues can be acute or chronic, resulting in different radiological appearances.

Acute periapical inflammatory change

Acute inflammation is generally a short-term situation, as the word means, in relation to disease, *coming sharply to a crisis*. The patient will have symptoms which will enable a diagnosis to be made and acted on; the radiographs may or may not provide any useful information. The only feature that can be expected to be evident is a widened periodontal ligament space which will be indistinguishable from that resulting from chronic occlusal forces. The presence or absence of infection will not influence this appearance. Failure to institute immediate treatment will result in the situation further progressing towards its crisis, or being modified by the body's healing response, into a chronic situation.

Chronic periapical inflammatory change

The majority of radiological changes result from chronic inflammation, and are influenced by patient factors, such as age, health, and virulence of the

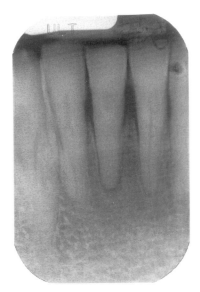

Fig. 7.6 Widened periodontal ligament space and loss of lamina dura of 41; there has also been obliteration of the pulp chamber by secondary dentine deposition. In the absence of caries, trauma or chronic occlusal forces are likely to have caused this early sign of inflammation. Note the two pulp canals in 42: M 53.

causative agent. The common appearances can be classified according to their description:

- Altered lamina dura
- Periapical radiolucency
- Periapical radiopacity
- Mixed radiolucency and opacity
- Root resorption
  - with no bone replacement
  - with bone replacement:
    normal
    opaque
- Exfoliation

Altered lamina dura

The lamina dura is the bony component of the periodontium (Sharpey fibre bone), and is the first part of the bone to be altered by the influences of chronic inflammation. The most important finding is loss of the lamina dura (Fig. 7.6), often interpreted as indicating that the tooth is non-vital. Unfortunately the demonstration of the lamina dura on a radiograph is not only dependent on its presence, but is strongly influenced by the radiographic projection, and exposure factors. Not seeing it does not mean that it is not there, whereas seeing it, does mean that it is there. Low-grade chronic inflammation can sometimes cause a thickening of the lamina dura rather than its depletion.

Periapical radiolucency

There are three possible explanations for inflammatory radiolucent changes:

1. Rarefying osteitis: non-specific destructive inflammatory change (Fig. 7.7). Frank infection is a feature of such change but is not always present. The margins may be well defined, but without a sclerotic margin, and the affected area of bone may be of variable size; the bone immediately adjacent may either be normal in appearance, or demonstrate increased opacity.

This description is applicable to teeth of the permanent dentition, and single-rooted teeth of the deciduous dentition. The inflammatory bone change in relation to two- and three-rooted deciduous teeth occurs in the inter-radicular area, as opposed to periapically, as the pulp is close to the periodontal ligament in this region in deciduous molars (Fig. 7.8).

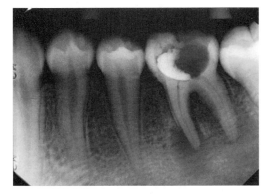

Fig. 7.7 Rarefying osteitis associated with both apices of 36. There is gross caries clearly involving the pulp chamber: M 14.

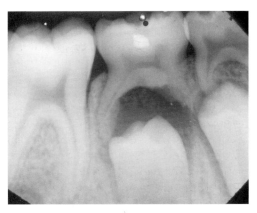

Fig. 7.8 Inter-radicular pattern of rarefying osteitis associated with deciduous molars: M 9.

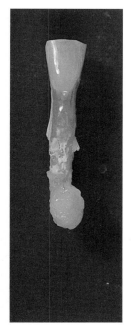

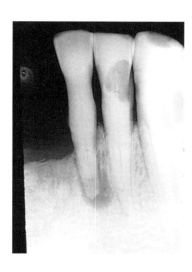

Fig. 7.9 Periapical granuloma attached to extracted 31 in an elderly man; the radiograph shows a completely sclerosed canal, and well defined, but non-corticated periapical radiolucency.

2. Periapical granuloma: Low-grade chronic inflammation of long standing is frequently manifested as a periapical granuloma. This chronic lesion is relatively avascular consisting mainly of fibroblasts. The opportunity to examine a clean lesion attached to an extracted tooth reveals a whitish, firm, spherical lesion, generally of a few millimetres diameter (Fig. 7.9). Radiologically such a lesion exhibits a relatively well-defined circular radiolucency which may or may not have a radiopaque margin. This appearance is characteristic of a benign, slow-growing, destructive lesion. The precise relationship to the apex of a tooth exhibiting features consistent with loss of vitality points to the diagnosis. Granulomata, of this kind, are always relatively small as the cells derive their nutrition by simple diffusion, and breakdown of the central zone will occur if the granuloma grows beyond a sustainable size. If this occurs epithelialization may follow with resultant cystic formation.

3. Periapical radicular cyst: These are inflammatory in origin, and arise as a result of proliferation of the epithelial cell rests of Malassez, found in the periodontal ligament (Fig. 7.10). They may arise *de novo*, or subsequent to a granuloma, as mentioned in the previous section. The classic radiological appearance of a radicular cyst is dealt with in Chapter 8.

Periapical radiopacity
Chronic inflammation is a balance between the destruction initiated by the abnormal irritant, and the reparative response by the involved and immediately adjacent tissues. The radiolucent changes described represent situations where the destructive aspect has the upper hand. In contrast, radiopaque changes indicate that the balance is in favour of the reparative agents, which, in bone, cause an increase in the mineral content of the bone. This situation is particularly seen in younger people, and is often associated with asymptomatic teeth. The radiological appearance represents *sclerosing osteitis* and is well demonstrated in Fig. 7.11. An increase in the radiopacity of the periapical or periradicular bone is not always attributable to a change in the status of

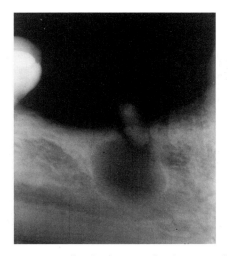

Fig. 7.10 Small radicular cyst related to apex of root fragment of 45: M 48

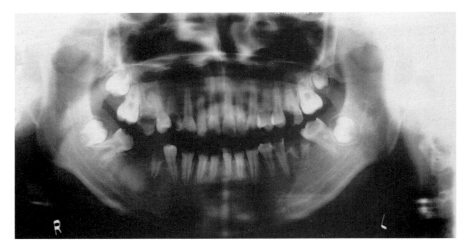

Fig. 7.11 Extensive asymptomatic caries has resulted in a variety of periapical inflammatory changes: sclerosing osteitis related to exfoliating distal root of 46; mesial root exfoliated completely; rarefying osteitis associated with 15, 35, and 45; exfoliating roots 36: F 14.

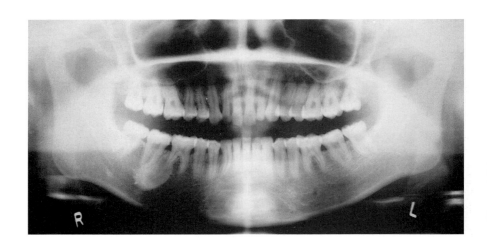

Fig. 7.12 Extensive sclerotic bone related to 46 and 47: both teeth are vital. Diagnosis: idiopathic osteosclerosis: F 18.

the pulp (Fig. 7.12), and a differential diagnosis of idiopathic osteosclerosis needs to be considered.

Mixed radiolucency and radiopacity
Rarefying and sclerosing osteitis can occur together, in the same patient, and in relation to the same tooth, or different teeth. When they occur in response to the same tooth they are always arranged with the radiolucent zone closest to the tooth, and the radiopaque zone closest to the remaining normal bone (Fig. 7.13).

Root resorption
The osteoclasts responsible for bone resorption are capable of resorbing roots. It is remarkable that in many situations there is no root resorption, in spite of extensive bone changes. When the roots are involved there is a variety of combinations that are depicted involving root and adjacent bone. The feature that is observed in each of these situations is that the root is shorter than expected, and the apex is blunter in appearance. Further examples of 'short roots' are discussed in Chapter 6, which considers the differential diagnosis of short roots.

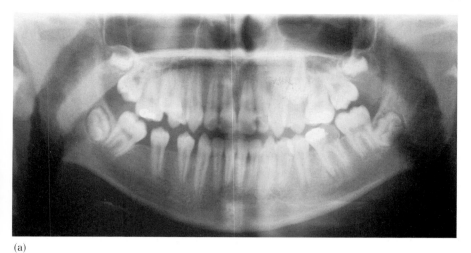

(a)

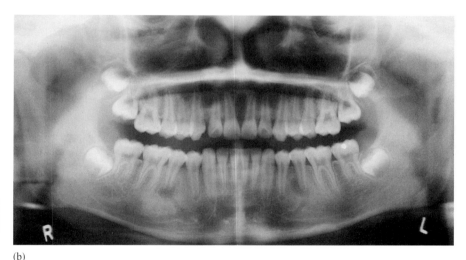

(b)

Fig. 7.13
(a) Sclerosing osteitis surrounding rarefying osteitis, related to 36: M 11.
(b) Sclerosing osteitis surrounding rarefying osteitis, related to open apices of non-vital 35 and 45; both teeth exhibit dens evaginatus; the open apices of the first premolars and second molars are due to normal root formation: M 14.

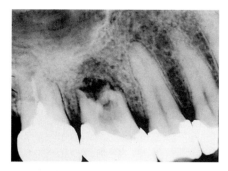

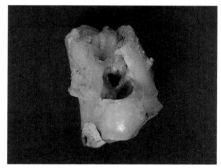

Fig. 7.14 Root resorption without bone replacement; the extracted tooth clearly shows the palatal cavity communicating with the pulp: M 37. The patient presented with a long history of discharge from the gingival crevice which had been treated unsuccessfully as a periodontal problem.

1. *Root resorption with no bone replacement*: when the inflammatory process is purely destructive the site previously occupied by the root remains radiolucent (Fig. 7.14).

2. *Root resorption with bone replacement*: in younger patients or those suffering from low-grade inflammation, the space left by the resorbed root may be filled in with alveolar bone. The bone may be normal in format and indistinguishable from the adjacent alveolar bone (Fig. 7.15), or exhibit evidence of sclerosing osteitis (Fig. 7.16).

Exfoliation
This is seen predominantly in young, healthy patients and is caused by the root continuing to erupt through the bone and gingival tissues, and ultimately being completely exfoliated (Fig. 7.11). The root maintains a completely

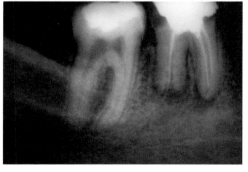

Fig. 7.15 Root resorption of both roots of 46 with replacement by normal bone; there is a separation zone between the apices and bone where active resorption is taking place. The endodontic therapy has not fully obliterated the pulp canals: F 27.

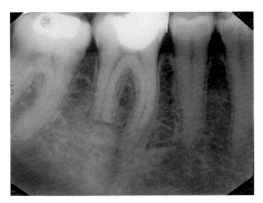

Fig. 7.16 Root resorption of distal root of 46 with replacement by sclerotic bone; the periapical bone related to the mesial root shows no evidence of inflammatory change: the mesial pulp may still be vital: M 29.

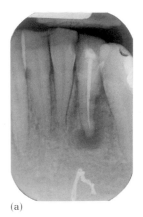
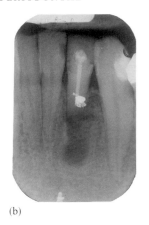
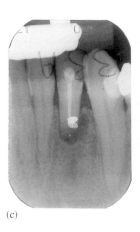

(a)   (b)   (c)

Fig. 7.17
(a) Root treated 32 with clear area of periapical inflammatory change: F 41.
(b) Immediately post-apicectomy.
(c) 14 months after the apicectomy there is complete healing of the periapical bone.

normal apical shape, unlike the blunt appearance seen when root resorption occurs. In order for this continued eruption to occur there has to be pre-existing destruction of the clinical crown.

Successful clinical treatment of periapical inflammatory pathology can result in complete resolution of the condition, and a return to normal, healthy bone. The case illustrated in Fig. 7.17 shows the result of apicectomy on a previously root-treated tooth; the patient had previously had an osteotomy, and there is evidence of a stainless steel wire in the first two images.

7.3.2   Periodontal

> *Periodontal*
>
> *peri*   = round, about.
> *odontos* = tooth.

The traditional concept of the periodontal structures are of those tissues involved in the support of the tooth; cementum, periodontal ligament, Sharpey fibre bone, inter-dental gingiva. The periapical region includes all these tissues, and forms a part of the periodontal support, but has been considered separately in view of the important link with the dental pulp.

Periodontal disease encompasses a collection of inflammatory disorders which affect the various components of the periodontium. Only changes to the supporting bone will be demonstrable radiologically. The most reliable information that can be obtained is the level of the bone on the mesial and distal aspects of a tooth, and the condition of the cortical bone forming the tooth socket and the alveolar crest. The bone level buccal and lingual to the roots cannot be identified due to the thin free margin coronally.

The bone level can be described as normal, exhibiting horizontal (regular) bone loss, or exhibiting vertical (irregular) bone loss. Any combination of these three is possible, such that there can be general or local areas of involvement. Both forms of bone loss can result from chronic inflammatory periodontal disease, and the expression is dependent on the virulence of the disease, and the resistance of the patient.

The normal, desirable, image is shown in Fig. 7.18. The cortical bone extending over the alveolar crest is not always so clearly shown, as its image will be influenced by projection geometry and exposure factors as well as its condition. The height of the alveolar margin relative to the enamel–root junction is influenced by the projection geometry of the radiographic technique:

(1) bisecting angle views will tend to cause an apparent improvement in buccal margins, and make lingual margins appear worse than they are;

(2) paralleling views, whether periapical or bitewing, will provide a more accurate impression of the true state of affairs.

Figure 7.19 illustrates the effect of altering vertical beam angulation on the apparent height of the bone margins.

(3) the panoramic radiograph has the advantage of employing the same projection geometry throughout the exposure, so that any distortion is standardized.

Calculus is radiopaque due to its calcium content, and can be detected on both the proximal surfaces of teeth, and when present in relation to the gingival margin (Fig. 7.20). In large quantities it can mask changes to the bone level, but should not result in confusion as it should be clearly evident clinically (see Fig. 6.19b).

Figures 7.21 to 7.26 are of a number of patients with varying expressions of periodontal disease, ranging from mild to a degree of severity in which it is remarkable that the teeth are still maintained by attachment to the soft tissues.

7.4 NON-INFLAMMATORY PATHOLOGICAL PERIAPICAL CHANGES

There are conditions which mimic inflammatory periapical pathology but which do not arise subsequent to pulpal or periodontal problems. They are less common than the inflammatory conditions, but are important as they emphasize the point that no assumption can be made about the state of the pulp of a tooth from its periapical appearance. Only one disorder, periapical cemental dysplasia, is likely to be mistaken for periapical inflammatory pathology, and

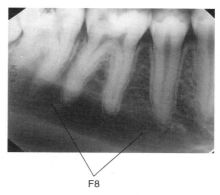

Fig. 7.18 Clear cortical bone forming the tooth sockets and interdental alveolar crests; caries in 46 and 47; marked radiolucency crossing the apices caused by the submandibular fossa below the mylohyoid ridge; 47 has 3 roots: F 17.

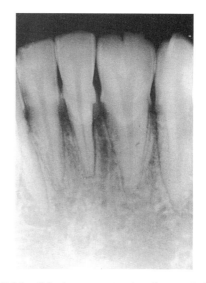

Fig. 7.20 Calculus on proximal surfaces and along the gingival margin of 31 and fused/geminated 32, forming radiopaque collars: M 26.

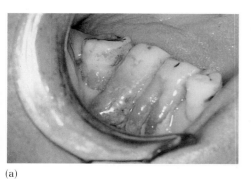
(a)

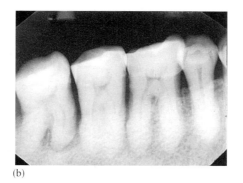
(b)

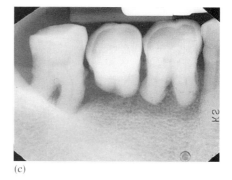
(c)

Fig. 7.19
(a) The clinical situation: 46 and 47 are lingually tilted and have no buccal bone support. (b) Vertical beam angulation at 90° to 46 and 47 gives the impression that they have adequate supporting bone.(c) Vertical beam angulation at 90° to 45 and 48 gives the true situation.

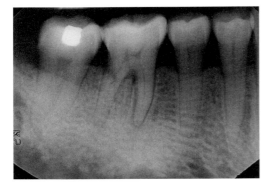

Fig. 7.21   Horizontal bone loss to furcation level; 46 is 3-rooted and surrounded by sclerotic bone: F 43.

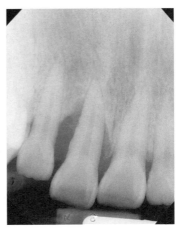

Fig. 7.22   Vertical bone loss related to 11: F 24.

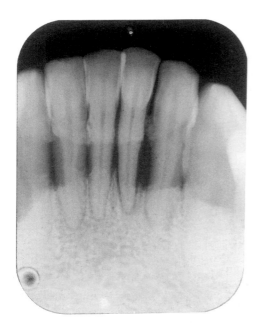

Fig. 7.23   Severe horizontal bone loss with extensive calculus deposits splinting the affected teeth.

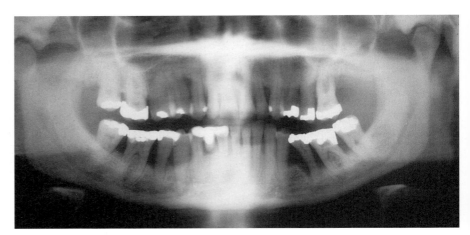

Fig. 7.24   Generalized horizontal bone loss, with vertical loss related to 35: F 45.

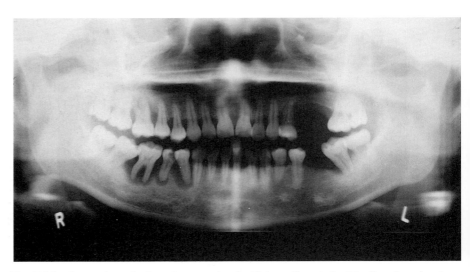

Fig. 7.25   Severe, irregular bone loss associated with juvenile periodontitis; there has already been loss of teeth as a result of the disease: F 21.

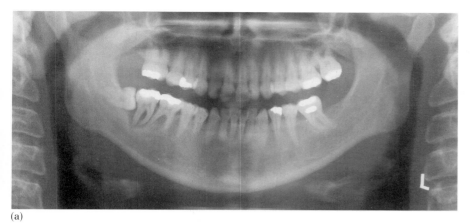

(a)

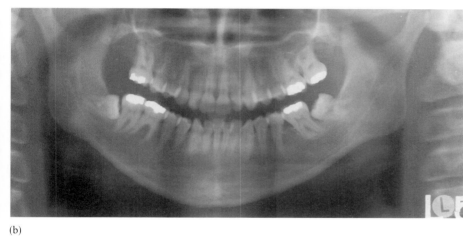

(b)

Fig. 7.26
(a) Perio-endo lesion related to 47 with severe vertical bone loss: F 31.
(b) 8 years previously there was no bone loss: the aetiological factor is the close proximity of 48: F 23.

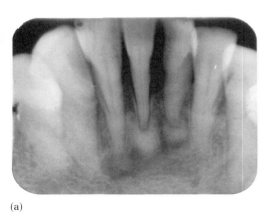

(a)

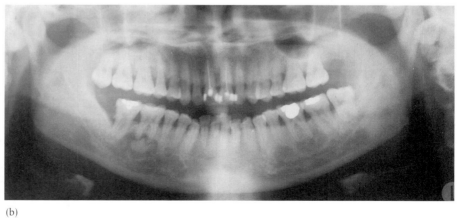

(b)

Fig. 7.27
(a) Multiple mixed radiolucent/radiopaque periapical lesions, with varying degrees of mineralization, due to periapical cemental dysplasia: F 57.
(b) Multiple mixed radiolucent/radiopaque periapical lesions associated with posterior teeth in mandible; all associated teeth vital; expected change in degree of radiopacity on radiographic follow up. Diagnosis: periapical cemental dysplasia: F 42.

is illustrated in Fig. 7.27. Other lesions that can also be described as periapical, but generally have additional distinguishing features, are mentioned in Chapters 8 and 9.

Periapical cemental dysplasia/osteofibrosis

This condition is most frequently seen in relation to the apices of lower incisors, and may affect multiple teeth. The initial appearance is of a discrete periapical radiolucency, not unlike that resulting from a granuloma. Over time, the lesion passes through a mixed radiolucent/radiopaque stage and ultimately manifests as a radiopacity. The vitality of involved teeth is not affected by these lesions.

8 Radiolucent lesions

8.1	INTRODUCTION	138
8.2	SITES AND MATERIALS INVOLVED	138
8.3	RADIOLUCENCIES	138
	8.3.1 Normal appearance and developmental variations	**139**
	8.3.2 Trauma	**139**
	8.3.3 Inflammatory	**139**
	8.3.4 Cystic	**139**
	8.3.5 Neoplastic	**144**
	8.3.6 Osteodystrophies	**145**
	8.3.7 Metabolic	**145**
	8.3.8 Idiopathic	**146**
	8.3.9 Iatrogenic	**146**
	8.3.10 Foreign bodies	**146**
	8.3.11 Artefacts	**146**

8   Radiolucent lesions

8.1   INTRODUCTION

The term 'radiolucent' is used to indicate that X-rays are penetrating a feature and that part of the film is then blackened. It can refer to absolute penetration as in the case of air, which has virtually no influence on the X-ray beam, or relative penetration with reference to the immediately adjacent feature. The most common use of the term 'radiolucent' applies when an isolated structure on the radiograph appears blacker than expected. This appearance is caused by either a reduction in total thickness, in the path of the X-ray beam, or a change in the nature of the material, such as the degree of mineralization.

At the kV levels that diagnostic dental X-ray machines operate at (50–100 kVp) absorption of X-rays is strongly dependent on the atomic number of the tissues and materials, being directly proportional to the cube of the atomic number (Chapter 1). The effect of this on the radiographic image is that even a relatively small change in the nature of a material will influence its X-ray absorption characteristics, and therefore radiological appearance.

The ultimate aim of examining radiographs is to link the information they provide with the patient's history, the symptoms, and the clinical findings, in order to arrive at a possible diagnosis. This is helped by using a 'radiological sieve' to prompt ideas. This was introduced in Chapter 3 and is reproduced in Appendix C.

8.2   SITES AND MATERIALS INVOLVED

Abnormal radiolucencies are most frequently detected in the hard tissues, that is the teeth and bony structures. Abnormalities which cause a change in soft tissues, or alter the contour of an air space, will only be detectable if there is sufficient difference in attenuating properties between them and the immediately adjacent feature. In practical terms, recognition of a radiolucency apparently within bone, is almost certain to be caused by a real change within the bone, rather than some other feature superimposed.

8.3   RADIOLUCENCIES

The examples used in this chapter have been selected to illustrate the relevance of the described features of a lesion. The categories of the radiological sieve will provide the framework, and a list of lesions that fall within each category will be provided, although not all will be illustrated. Radiolucencies affecting the crown of the tooth, inflammatory periapical lesions, and lesions resulting from trauma are illustrated in Chapters 5, 7, and 10, respectively. In addition, there are examples elsewhere in the text of many of the lesions listed.

The description of each example will include the features of the *detailed examination*, in descriptive form, in order to provide a mental picture of the lesion, and enable comparison with other radiolucencies. The *impression* that is given by the combination of features will be discussed, and the provisional or differential diagnosis provided, with the follow-up and actual diagnosis where this is relevant.

8.3.1   Normal appearance and developmental variations

A number of examples of the appearance of normal structures, and their appearance during development are provided in earlier chapters. For the purpose of later comparisons two features are illustrated here: the developing tooth germ (Figs 8.1 and 8.2), and the cleft palate (Fig. 8.3).

8.3.2   Trauma

Traumatic injuries to the teeth are illustrated in Chapter 10.

8.3.3   Inflammatory

Examples of caries, root resorption, and rarefying osteitis are provided elsewhere. It is important to be aware of the possibility of existing lesions becoming secondarily infected, and how their appearance becomes altered. Figures 8.4 and 8.5 illustrate primary and secondary infection.

8.3.4   Cystic

A cyst is an epithelial-lined, fluid-filled pathological lesion. Cysts may occur within bone and soft tissue; in the jaws, cysts may be odontogenic or non-odontogenic in origin, and account for the majority of radiolucent lesions of notable size (Figs 8.6–8.17).

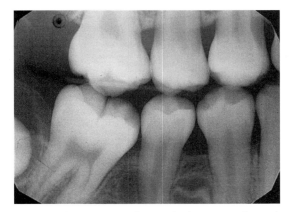

Fig. 8.1   M 15, presenting for routine check-up. *Film*: bitewing radiograph.
Two circular, well-defined radiolucencies in the right body of the mandible, approximately 5 mm in diameter, with radiopaque margins: one is partially superimposed on the root of 45, and distal to it; the second is between 44 and 45, and contains a radiopaque line in the form of twin peaks: the related teeth have normal images.
Impression: the appearance of the radiolucencies is typical of early tooth formation, prior to calcification, and shortly after it has commenced.
Provisional diagnosis: late-developing supplemental premolars.

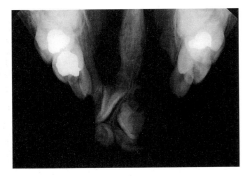

Fig. 8.3   M 5, bilateral cleft palate, attending for check-up.
Film: upper anterior oblique occlusal.
This child was known to have a cleft palate which had been diagnosed at birth. The radiograph demonstrates the lack of bone bilaterally lateral to the premaxilla; 12 is present but 22 is absent, and there is malformation of the developing 21.

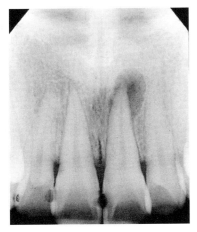

Fig. 8.4   F 20, asymptomatic.
Film: periapical.
Well-defined oval lesion related to apex of 21; approximately 6 mm diameter with radiopaque margin; radiolucencies in 12 m, 11 m, and 21 m involving enamel and dentine.
Impression: caries or unlined radiolucent restorations in 12, 11, and 21; periapical inflammatory lesion associated with 21, secondary to loss of vitality.
Differential diagnosis (of periapical lesion): periapical granuloma; radicular cyst.
Follow-up: check vitality of 21; endodontic treatment; radiographic review; apicectomy if no resolution of lesion.

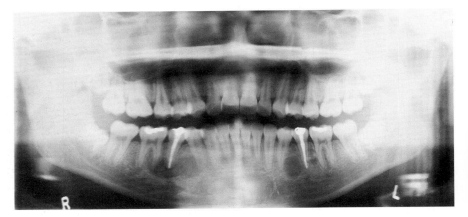

Fig. 8.2   F 14, Chinese, presenting for routine check-up, no symptoms.*Film*: panoramic radiograph.Four areas of radiolucency, two in each body of the mandible: (a) Between and superimposed on 35 and 36, well defined, with internal calcification, no effect on adjacent structures. (b) Oval, well-defined lesion with radiopaque margin between 34 and 35, just over-lapping 34 but otherwise not apparently related to either tooth; 35 has been root-treated; the roots of 34 and 35 are further apart at the apices than coronally; (c) Oval lesion between 44 and 45, similar to (b), except that the margins are rather diffuse and it is less clearly radiolucent; the roots of 44 and 45 are similar to 34 and 35; (d) Oval (long axis horizontal) lesion encom-passing 45 apex and mesial apex of 46, diffuse margin; 45 has been root-treated.
Impression: the lack of clarity of the lesions on the right is more likely due to the panoramic tech-nique than the lesions, as all the teeth in this section are slightly blurred; 35 and 36 were proba-bly Leung's premolars, and became non-vital as a result of traumatic damage to the pulp; the lesion between 35 and 36 has the characteristics of a developing tooth germ, and therefore all the lesions may be similar; the lesion associated with the apices of 45 and 46 may be inflamma-tory in origin, caused by non-vital 45.
Differential diagnosis: developing supernumerary tooth germs; periapical inflammatory lesion (45/46).
Follow-up: radiography in 1 year unless signs or symptoms suggestive of infection develop.

The cysts listed below are those most frequently seen within the jaws, and are named here in accordance with the World Health Organisation classification (Figs 8.6–8.18).

Odontogenic

Radicular: this inflammatory cyst arises in relation to the root of a tooth; if the tooth is removed and the cyst left behind then it is termed residual.

Paradental: histologically, this is identical to the radicular cyst, but radiologi-cally it is often related to the crown and root of a partially erupted tooth.

Dentigerous: arises from the follicle of an erupted tooth, and displaces the tooth as it expands, maintaining an attachment to the neck of the tooth.

Eruption: arises from the follicle of an erupting tooth, which may then erupt normally as the result of interventional or traumatic marsupialization of the cyst (see Fig. 5.16).

Keratocyst: arises from the dental lamina or its remnants, not in relation to a tooth, although not infrequently there is an intimate relationship with an unerupted tooth, mimicking a dentigerous cyst.

Calcifying odontogenic: a true cyst containing varying amounts of radiopaque material.

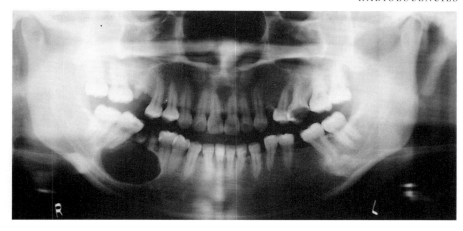

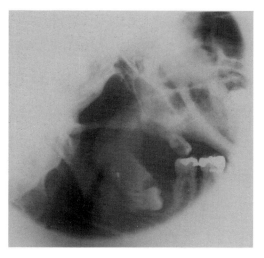

Fig. 8.6 F 21, complaining of painless swelling right mandible.
Film: panoramic radiograph.
There is a large (3 × 2 cm), oval, well-defined radiolucency in the right body of the mandible, with a radiopaque margin, associated with retained root fragments from grossly carious 46; there is displacement of 47 and the ID canal.
Impression: a benign, long-established, slowly expanding cystic lesion, aetiologically related to 46.
Provisional diagnosis: radicular cyst associated with 46.
Follow-up: enucleation and removal of 46 roots.

Fig. 8.5 M 54, presented complaining of pain and swelling in region of lower right third molar.
Film: oblique lateral of right ramus.
The follicular space associated with unerupted, horizontally impacted 48 shows an increase in size, with diffuse margins; the tooth appears to be displaced infero-posteriorly; its roots overlap the image of the ID canal which is unaltered. There are radiolucencies in the crowns of 17 (18) and 47 m, and a small radiopaque area just above the ID canal near the lingula.
Impression: enlargement of the follicle of 48 and loss of definition of the crypt outline due to inflammation; the size is suggestive of underlying cystic transformation; caries in 17 and 47; foreign body or artefact causing radiopacity. (See Fig. 9.18.)
Differential diagnosis: infected dentigerous cyst associated with 48; infected follicle of 48.
Follow-up: (1) treat the infection; (2) remove 48 together with the associated soft tissue; (3) optional histopathological examination.

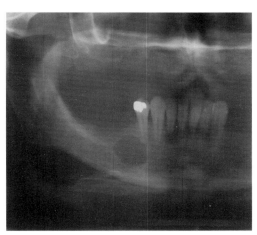

Fig. 8.7 M 33, irregular attender, complaining of symptoms related to lower incisors.
Film: sectional panoramic.
Only 7 teeth are remaining with radiolucent lesions related to 2.
(a) An almost circular lesion in the right body of the mandible, approximately 1.5 cm diameter, with a well-defined, radiopaque margin; asymmetrically related to apex of 45, the margin is continuous with socket outline; relation to ID canal unclear.
(b) A periapical circular lesion associated with 42, approximately 6 mm diameter, well-defined but not radiopaque margin; there appears to be apical root resorption of 42. However, careful examination, blocking out all extraneous light and masking the image to the relevant portion, demonstrates that the apex is present, and it is the severe bone loss that is causing difficulty in visualizing it.
Impression: two different but probably inflammatory lesions in this poorly cared for mouth:
(a) is benign, established, and cystic in appearance; 45 is heavily restored but not centrally placed in the lesion;
(b) exhibits signs of active inflammation and may be a perio-endo lesion in view of the alveolar bone loss; there is no caries or restoration in the tooth.
Differential diagnosis:
(a) residual cyst 46, radicular cyst 45;
(b) periapical granuloma, rarefying osteitis.

Fig. 8.8a   F 26, chance finding after taking panoramic radiograph.

Film: oblique occlusal radiograph.

A well-defined pear-shaped lesion involving the apices of 32–42, with a sclerotic margin; coronal radiolucencies in 31, 41, and 42; periodontal ligament space evident around 32, 31, and 42.

Impression: a benign lesion which may or may not be odontogenic in origin; the radiolucencies in the crowns of the teeth are relatively small carious lesions, and there are no symptoms.

Differential diagnosis: radicular cyst; solitary bone cyst; radiographic artefact due to symphyseal architecture.

Follow-up: vitality test of 41 was negative; the tooth must have become non-vital in relation to trauma.

Fig. 8.8b   The tooth was endodontically treated, and apicectomy and enucleation carried out; histology, radicular cyst.

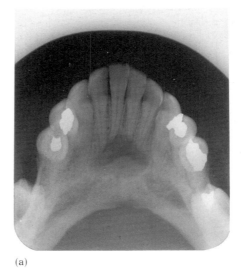 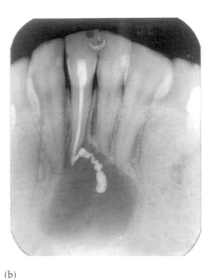

(a)   (b)

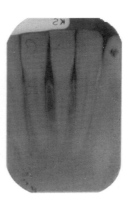

Fig. 8.9   M 22, complaining of pain and swelling lower anterior region.

Films: periapicals of 32–42, and lower anterior oblique occlusal

(a) A diffuse radiolucency related to the lower incisors, full extent not clear (on periapicals); the teeth appear sound. The lesion's presence and margins are even more unclear on the lower anterior oblique occlusal.

Impression: radiologically the diffuse nature of the lesion, associated with apparently normal teeth indicates the possibility of a solitary bone cyst or cemento-osseous dysplasia, rather than an inflammatory lesion.

Differential diagnosis: solitary bone cyst; cemento-osseous dysplasia; radicular cyst; keratocyst.

Follow-up: vitality tests revealed 41 and 42 non-vital: this puts periapical inflammatory bone change to the top of the list, and endodontic treatment is indicated; a biopsy was taken which determined a histological diagnosis of radicular cyst.

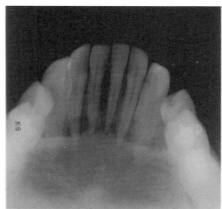

Non-odontogenic

Nasopalatine duct cyst: arises in the midline of the maxilla.

Solitary bone cyst: a non-epithelialized 'cystic' cavity, which can mimic other cystic lesions: the diagnosis is usually clear at surgery when no epithelial lining can be found.

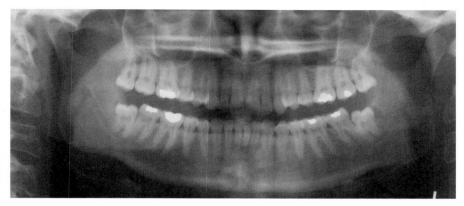

Fig. 8.10   F 22, referred for investigation of third molars.
Film: panoramic.
Crescent-shaped radiolucent lesion associated with distal aspect of crown and root of partially
erupted, disto-angular 38; approximately 1 × 0.5 cm, with well-defined and radiopaque margin.
Impression: a benign cystic lesion, likely to be of odontogenic origin; the clarity of the margins
indicates that there is no active inflammation.
Differential diagnosis: paradental cyst; dentigerous cyst.
Follow-up: 38 is not going to erupt into a functional position and is therefore extracted;
histopathological examination indicated a diagnosis of paradental cyst.

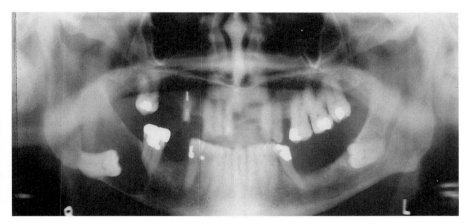

Fig. 8.11   M 71, referred for full examination and treatment planning.
Film: panoramic.
Extensive radiolucent lesion extending from mesial of 47 to level with lingula, predominantly but
not exclusively above ID canal; well-defined lesion with sections of the margin radiopaque;
enclosing the crown and part of the root of displaced 48; the ID canal has been displaced
inferiorly.
Impression: a benign cystic lesion, expanding slowly and causing displacement of other
structures, which may have arisen from 48 follicle.
Provisional diagnosis: dentigerous cyst associated with 48.
Follow-up: surgical enucleation of the cyst and removal of 48 allowed histopathological
verification of the diagnosis.

Aneurysmal bone cyst: a 'cystic' lesion comprising blood-filled spaces, and
varying degrees of fibroblastic tissue, osteoid, and woven bone.

*The pathological lesions listed in the remaining sections are not described here, as
their pathology and aetiology is well covered in other texts listed in the
Bibliography. The lesions that are illustrated, in order to assist with the differential
diagnosis of radiolucent lesions, are marked with an asterisk (*).*

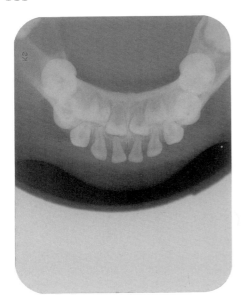
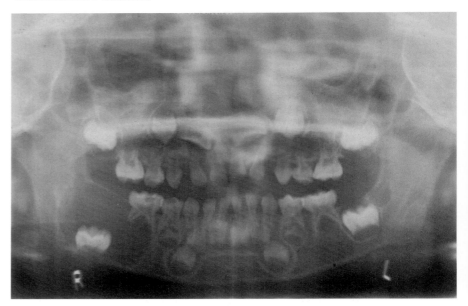

Fig. 8.12   M 3, parents concerned about increasing facial asymmetry.
Films: panoramic and lower true occlusal.
Well-defined, corticated radiolucency in right body of mandible, encompassing crown of developing 46 and extending from mesial of 85 to lingula region of ramus; resorption of the distal root of 85 is evident; the ID canal is not visible right or left.
Impression: a benign, slow-growing cystic lesion, probably arising from the follicle of 46.
Provisional diagnosis: dentigerous cyst associated with 46.
Follow-up: marsupialisation of the cyst encourages the affected tooth to erupt towards the occlusal plane; enucleation would result in the loss of 85, 46, 45, and 47.

8.3.5   Neoplastic

Tumours are customarily divided into benign and malignant lesions, on the basis of the propensity for metastasizing; the ameloblastoma falls between these two groups as it can be locally very aggressive, but does not metastasize. The appearance of ameloblastomas can be very varied, and therefore a selection of cases will be illustrated, in addition to the presentation of malignant radiolucent lesions. The other lesions listed here and in other texts, occur less frequently; their management will be influenced by the radiological appearance they present, whether or not there is a label attached in terms of a possible diagnosis. (Figs 8.19–8.22 and 8.24–8.26).

Benign lesions

- Ameloblastoma*
- Pindborg tumour (calcifying epithelial odontogenic tumour)
- Fibroma
- Myxoma
- Neurilemmoma
- Haemangioma*
- Melanotic neuro-ectodermal tumour of infancy*

Malignant lesions

- Carcinomas, primary* and secondary
- Non-osteogenic osteosarcoma

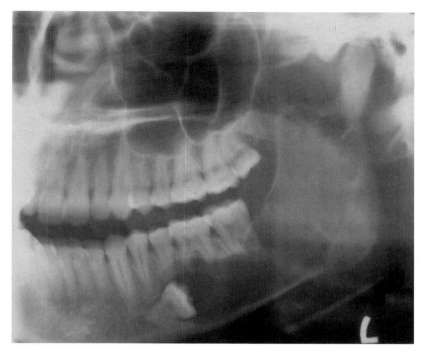

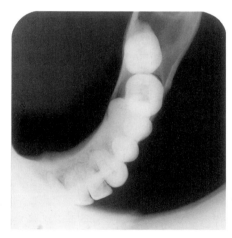

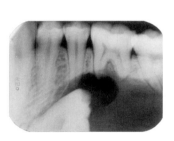

Fig. 8.13 F 24, complained of altered sensation over distribution of left ID nerve.
Films: panoramic (Panorex), bisecting angle periapical and left lower true occlusal.
Extensive, well-defined radiolucent lesion involving a large part of the left body and ramus, extending from 35 to the sigmoid notch; the margin is generally corticated and loculated in places; 38 has been displaced to the anterior aspect of the lesion with its crown within the lesion; there is no expansion, but perforation bucally; the ID canal has been displaced inferiorly; there is root resorption affecting 36.
Impression: this is a long-standing cystic lesion giving conflicting messages: the relation to 38 indicates a dentigerous cyst; the cortical perforation and root resorption suggests an aggressive lesion; the multi-locularity is suggestive of uneven growth, and the loss of sensation is suspicious.
Differential diagnosis: keratocyst; dentigerous cyst. Ameloblastoma is not considered as there is no expansion.
Follow-up: the lesion was biopsied and proved to be a keratocyst.

- Multiple myeloma*
- Histiocytosis X

8.3.6 Osteodystrophies

- Fibrous dysplasia
- Cherubism
- Early Paget's disease of bone
- Periapical cemental dysplasia/osteofibrosis* (See Chapter 7)
- Early ossifying/cementifying fibroma*

8.3.7 Metabolic

- Central giant cell granuloma* (hyperparathyroidism)
- Vitamin deficiencies

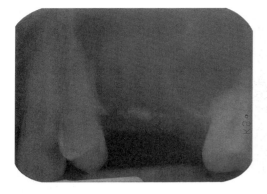

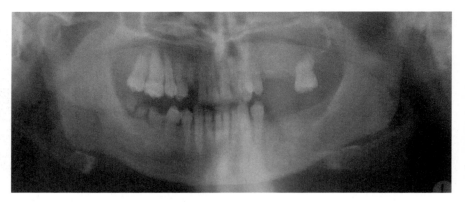

Fig. 8.14 M 41, complaining of pain in left upper jaw, and large soft tissue mass bucally; symptoms commenced 2 years previously.
Films: panoramic, OM, and periapical 23–27.
In the left maxillary alveolus extending posteriorly from the distal aspect of 24, and superiorly into the antrum is an extensive radiolucent lesion, with a variable margin; in the lowest portion of the lesion there are a number of small discrete radiopacities, of a similar opacity to dentine. The size of the lesion, and the involvement of the maxillary antrum make a judgement of precise size and shape difficult; there is destruction of the lateral wall of the antrum, and a faint image of the expansile lesion close to the left coronoid process.
Impression: a destructive, expansile lesion, expanding more rapidly than the pace of bony remodelling, with evidence of internal calcification.
Differential diagnosis: calcifying epithelial odontogenic cyst; Pindborg tumour; (infected) odontogenic keratocyst.
Follow-up: histology, after excisional biopsy, indicated that the lesion was an odontogenic keratocyst; calcification is unusual and indicative of chronic inflammation over a period of time.

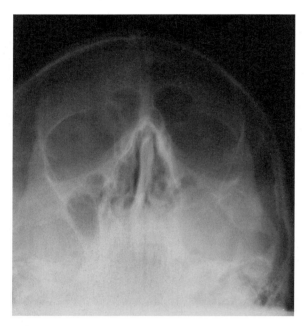

- Osteoporosis

8.3.8   Idiopathic

- Stafne idiopathic bone cavity* (Fig. 8.29)

8.3.9   Iatrogenic

- Restorations
- Damage during dental treatment: restorative or surgical

8.3.10   Foreign bodies

- Non-opaque objects, e.g. beads

8.3.11   Artefacts

- Cervical radiolucency (See Chapter 5)
- Handling and chemical artefacts

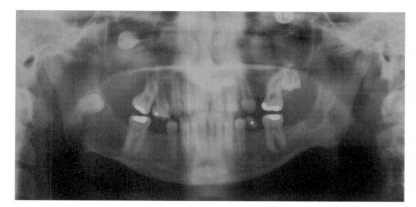

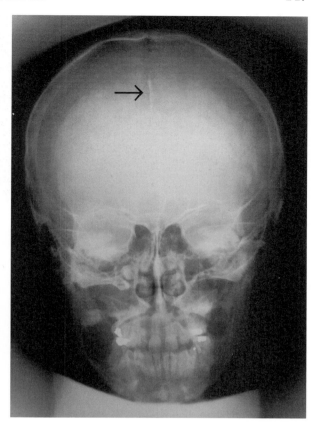

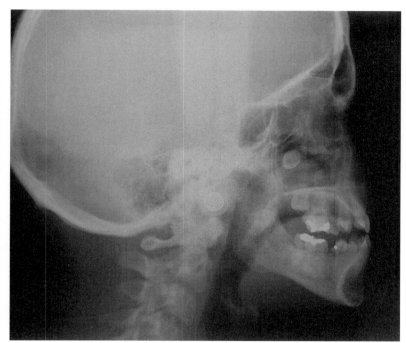

Fig. 8.15   F 16, original referral to investigate presence of third molars, with subsequent additional radiography.
Films: panoramic, PA mandible, lateral ceph.
There are three separate radiolucent lesions, one in each quadrant except the second; on the right the lesions are associated with unerupted third molars; no dental involvement is evident on the left; the involved teeth are displaced. In the maxilla, the lesion has involved the maxillary sinus and the appearance is therefore relatively radiopaque; each lesion has a smooth, well-defined outline, the mandibular lesions exhibit cortication.

Each lesion is a different size and their effect on other structures varies in relation to this:
(a) Upper right is approximately 3.5 cm diameter, and has displaced 18 which is high in the maxilla, relatively medial with its crown facing laterally.
(b) Lower left is approximately 1 cm diameter and superficially placed with no effect on other structures.
(c) Lower right is approximately 3.5 cm antero-posteriorly and has displaced the ID canal inferiorly.

The PA view demonstrates a linear calcification in the midline (arrowed) superimposed on the sagittal suture: the position and extent is in accordance with a calcified falx cerebri.
Impression: the concurrent presentation of multiple cystic radiolucencies, and a calcified falx suggests a diagnosis of multiple keratocysts, as part of a more widespread syndrome.
Provisional diagnosis: multiple keratocysts, associated with multiple naevoid basal cell carcinoma and jaw cyst syndrome. In view of the likelihood of this diagnosis the patient should undergo a thorough examination in order to ascertain the presence of other associated anomalies.

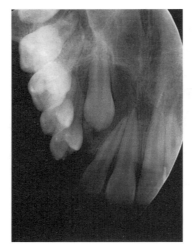
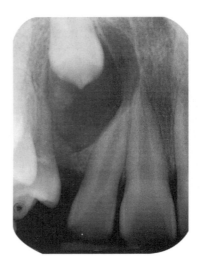

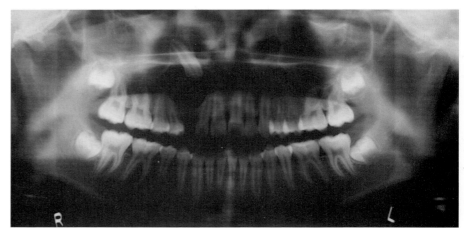

Fig. 8.16 M 15, investigated for unerupted upper right canine.

Films: panoramic, upper oblique occlusal and periapical (both centred on 13).

13 is high up in the maxilla and associated with a circular radiolucent lesion of approximately 2.5 cm diameter, having a well-defined corticated margin, extending between the apices of 11 and 15, and containing a small amount of radiopaque material close to the crown of 13; there appears to be some tipping of the related teeth.

Impression: a benign, relatively slow-growing cystic lesion, probably odontogenic in origin. The changing relations of the lesion and 13 between the films indicates that the bulk of the lesion is palatal to 13.

Differential diagnosis: odontogenic keratocyst; dentigerous cyst; calcifying epithelial odontogenic cyst; globulo-maxillary cyst.

Follow-up: excisional biopsy proved that 13 and the cystic lesion were separate; the lesion was diagnosed as a calcifying epithelial odontogenic cyst.

Fig. 8.17 F 40, follow-up after apicectomy of 21 and 23.

Film: upper anterior oblique occlusal. There is a midline circular radiolucency of 11 mm diameter with a well-defined corticated margin; 11, 21, and 23 have been endodontically treated and apicectomies with retrograde amalgams carried out on 21 and 23; there are clear periodontal ligament spaces around the incisor apices; fragments of markedly radiopaque material are within the lesion.

Impression: the initial impression in relation to obviously non-vital teeth is that this must be a radicular cyst. However, the clear periodontal ligament space contradicts this, and favours a non-odontogenic lesion.

Differential diagnosis: radicular cyst (see impression); nasopalatine duct cyst; enlarged but normal nasopalatine duct.

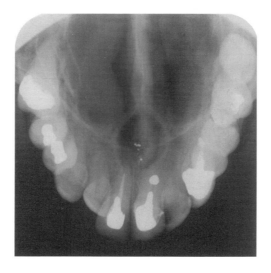

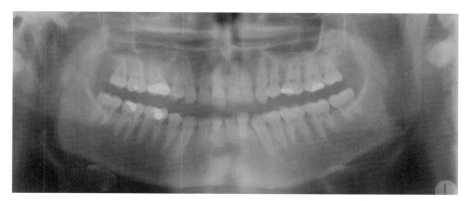

Fig. 8.18 M 20

Film: panoramic.

There is an irregular shaped radiolucent lesion in the left body of the mandible, extending from the mesial root of 36 to the distal root of 37, and from just below the alveolar crest to below the ID canal; approximately 3 × 2.5 cm, it has well-defined margins which are radiopaque in parts; it extends up between the roots of 36 and 37; the associated teeth appear to be healthy; there is also a small denticle between 32 and 33, better seen on a periapical.

Impression: a cystic lesion with no apparent aetiological source.

Differential diagnosis: if the teeth concerned are vital: solitary bone cyst; a cemento-osseous lesion; odontogenic keratocyst. If the teeth are non-vital: radicular cyst.

Follow-up: the lesion was explored and proved to have no epithelial lining: a diagnosis of solitary bone cyst was made on the basis of this finding and the non-specific contents of the bone cavity. Such surgical exploration is usually sufficient to initiate healing of these cavities.

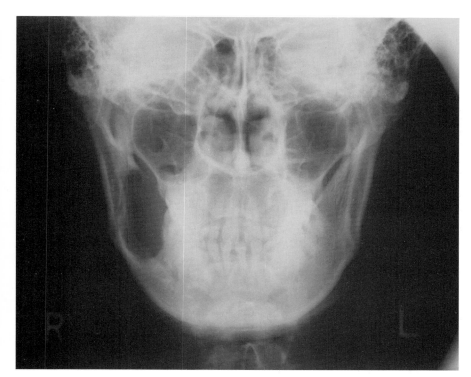

Fig. 8.19 F 20, complaining of pain and swelling right posterior mandible.

Films: panoramic and PA mandible. There is a large radiolucent lesion involving right angle of mandible, extending from mesial root of 47 to height of lingula, and involving all bone superficial to the ID canal; kidney-shaped, it is approximately 6 × 4 cm; the lower border is well defined and corticated; the upper border is extra-bony and not evident; the medial border is demarcated by a very thin bony covering which has been expanded; the distal root of 47 is within the lesion, and has a blunt apex; the ID canal runs along the lower border of the lesion at a lower level than on the left. The mouth is unrestored and caries-free.

Impression: an aggressive but relatively slow-growing (ID canal displacement) destructive (47 root resorption) lesion, possibly of odontogenic origin; neoplastic or cystic.

Differential diagnosis: ameloblastoma; odontogenic keratocyst; giant cell lesion.

Note the retained 62 related to the bimaxillary anterior spacing; peg-shaped upper lateral incisors; sclerotic bone related to the mesial root of 36.

Follow-up: excisional biopsy and removal of 47 was carried out; the histological diagnosis was ameloblastoma

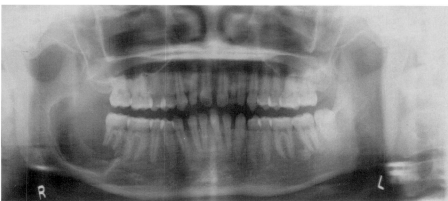

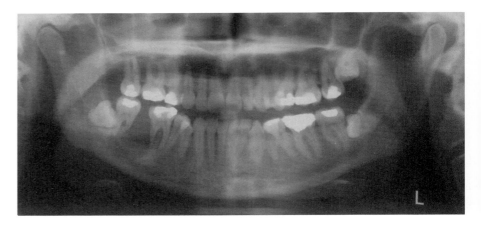

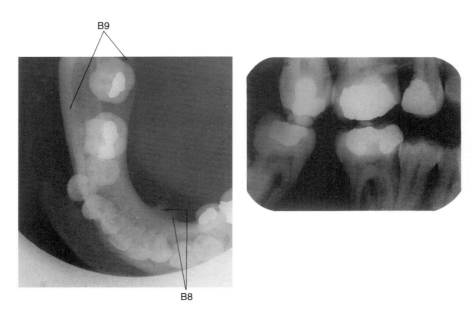

Fig. 8.20 F 33, referred for further investigation after chance finding of unusual radiolucency on bitewing radiograph.

Films: panoramic, bitewing, and true occlusal.

There is a radiolucent unilocular lesion in the right body of mandible, related to 46 and 47 and extending from the alveolar crest to the ID canal; it is almost circular with a diameter of approximately 2 cm; the margins are ill defined, blending into the surrounding bone; the distal root of 46 and the mesial root of 47 are involved in, and separated by, the lesion; the lesion extends to but does not involve the upper border of the ID canal; 46 is quite heavily restored; 47 is restored but there is no evidence of pulpal involvement; the true occlusal view shows that the lesion has expanded lingually and has perforated the cortical bone; there is possible resorption of the distal root of 46.

Impression: a rapidly advancing destructive lesion, which may or may not be odontogenic in origin, but requires urgent investigation to determine its true nature.

Differential diagnosis: giant cell lesion; infected radicular cyst; ameloblastoma; odontogenic keratocyst; cemento-osseous lesion.

  Excisional biopsy determined a diagnosis of unilocular cystic ameloblastoma.

  The tiny radiopaque marks on the true occlusal view buccal to the mandible are caused by pressure marks.

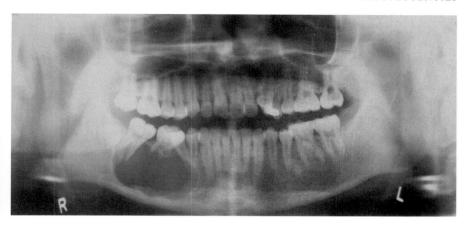

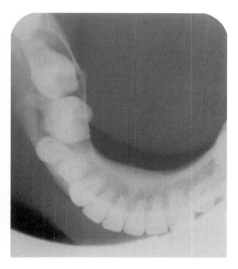

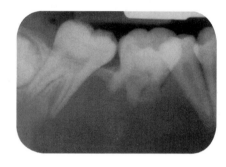

Fig. 8.21   M 15, referred for investigation of non-painful expansion of right mandible.
Films: panoramic, lower true occlusal, and periapical.
A well-defined, partially corticated radiolucency involving the right body of the mandible from 44 to 47 distal; the ID canal is displaced inferiorly and there is tipping of related teeth; lingual expansion with cortical thinning and buccal expansion with destruction of the cortex (it can only be seen with added masking); shortening of the roots of 46.
Impression: an aggressive, fast-growing, locally destructive lesion, most likely to be neoplastic.
Follow-up: biopsy provided a histological diagnosis of cystic ameloblastoma.

The order of examination of the radiographs, leading to the descriptions provided in the captions, is covered in detail in Chapter 3 and Appendix C; an explanation of the relevance of each descriptive feature can be found in the named sections.

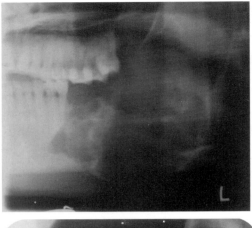

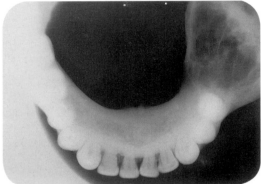

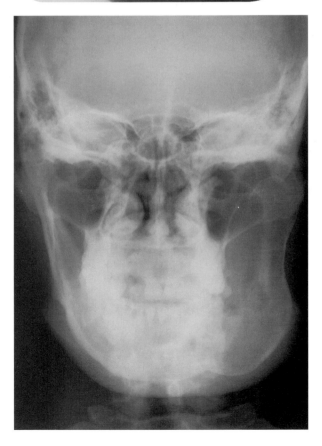

Fig. 8.22   M 24, self-referred for treatment of massive expansion of left side of face; 3 teeth had been extracted in his home country to no effect.
Films: panoramic, lower true occlusal, and PA mandible.
Massive soap-bubble radiolucent lesion involving the whole of the left ramus and the body up to 34; the expansion is in every direction and the cortex is thin but intact; the ID canal is displaced to the lower margin of the mandible but is still centrally positioned (occlusal view); the socket of recently extracted 38 is evident.
Impression: a long-standing benign lesion with considerable growth potential, cystic or neoplastic, odontogenic or non-odontogenic.
Differential diagnosis: aneurysmal bone cyst; ameloblastoma.
Follow-up: biopsy provided a histological diagnosis of ameloblastoma; the mandible was resected in view of the size of the lesion.

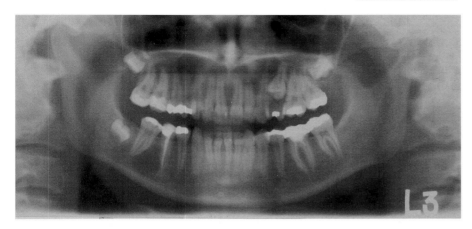

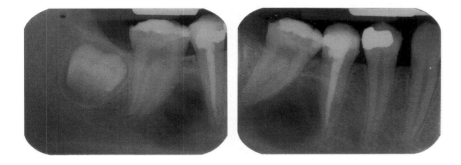

Fig. 8.23   F 15, complaining of dull ache in lower right quadrant, short history; clinically there was no expansion.
Films: panoramic and periapicals.
There is a circular radiolucency in the right body of the mandible mainly between 45 and 47 (46 has been previously extracted), partially
superimposed on the root of 45, extending from 4 mm below the crest of the ridge to the lower border of the ID canal; the margins are well defined but not corticated; 45 has been
endodontically treated; there is no clear lamina dura on 45 distal or 47 mesial; the ID canal is at the same level as the canal on the left.
Impression: a benign, expansile lesion, probably odontogenic in origin, most likely to be an infected residual cyst (from 46).
Differential diagnosis: residual cyst (46); (lateral) radicular cyst (45); solitary bone cyst; keratocyst; fibroma; unicystic ameloblastoma.
Follow-up: the lesion was enucleated and found to have no epithelial lining; the soft tissue contents of the bony cavity were friable, and predominantly vascular dense connective tissue, and woven bone. A histological diagnosis of primary intra-osseous haemangioma *or* solitary bone cyst was made.

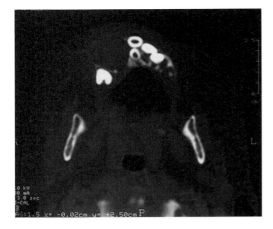

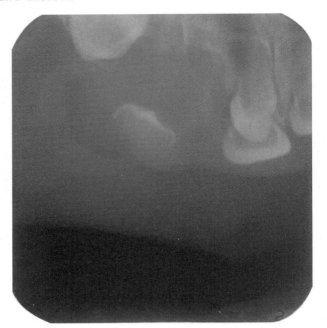

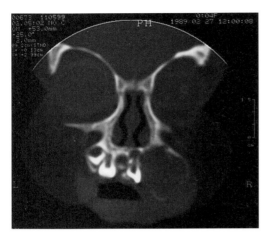

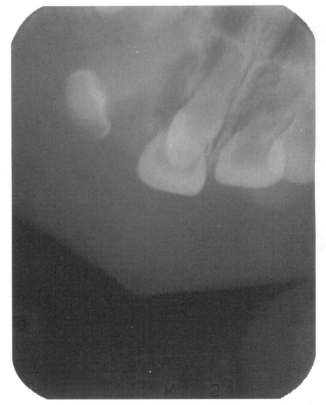

Fig. 8.24 F 4 months old, presented with rapidly expanding lesion in right maxilla, and related difficulties in feeding; otherwise well, and not distressed.
Films: two oblique occlusals, and CT scans.
There is a marked radiolucency involving the majority of the right maxilla, with obvious displacement of all the associated developing teeth. The margins are diffuse on the intra-oral films, but well demarcated on the CT scans.
Impression: a rapid, destructive, but contained tumorous growth.
Reproduced with kind permission of Butterworth-Heinemann (DMFR, 1991, Vol. 20, 172–4).
Follow-up: the lesion was biopsied and histologically diagnosed as a melanotic neuro-ectodermal tumour of infancy. Local excision was performed and no subsequent recurrence

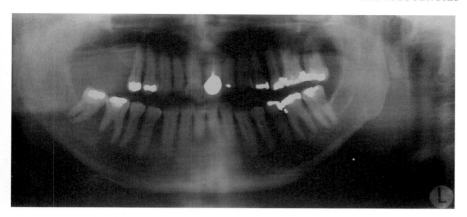

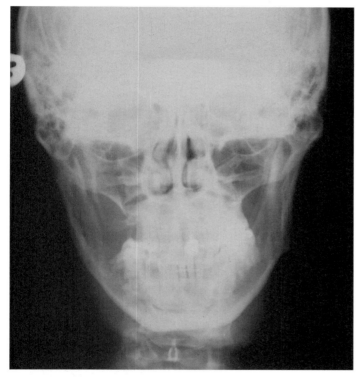

Fig. 8.25   M 54, complaining of non-healing ulcer lingual to right posterior mandible.
Films: panoramic and PA mandible.
There is diffuse patchy alteration in bone pattern of the right ramus of the mandible, and the
body distal to 46; the PA mandible gives a clearer impression of the involvement which particularly affects the lingual aspect; the margins are unclear and there is destruction of the lingual
cortex with no suggestion of attempts to repair; the roots of 47 and distal root of 46 are involved
in the altered bone; these teeth are restored but there is no
evidence of pulpal involvement; in addition to the lingual cortical destruction there is thinning of
the cortical bone of the inferior border of the mandible; the ID canal does not show clearly on
either side.
Impression: a non-uniform destructive lesion, with no evidence of associated repair, neoplastic or
infective in origin.
Differential diagnosis: squamous cell carcinoma; severe osteomyelitis. The other aspects of the
examination are critical in determining whether this is most likely to be neoplastic or
inflammatory. This case illustrates how subtle the bone changes can be in certain views, which
increases the risk of their being missed. Radiologically, there is little difference between a primary
and a secondary carcinoma in bone: if a primary there will be obvious clinical involvement.
Follow-up: biopsy provided a histological diagnosis of squamous cell carcinoma.

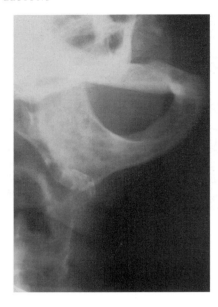

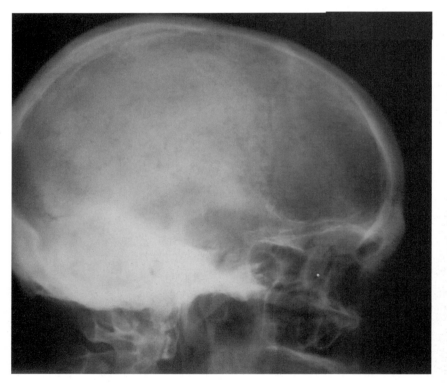

Fig. 8.26   M 71
Films: oblique lateral mandible and lateral skull.
There are widespread, multiple discrete 'punched-out' radiolucencies in the bones of the skull vault and mandible; the circular lesions are approximately 2–3 mm diameter, well defined, but not corticated, with no particular relation to other structures.
Impression: a widespread disorder, either systemic in origin, or neoplastic; the 'punched-out' appearance of the radiolucencies occurring in multiple bones is strongly suggestive of multiple myeloma.
Provisional diagnosis: multiple myeloma.
The diagnosis was confirmed on biopsy.

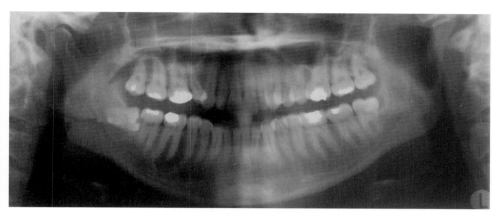

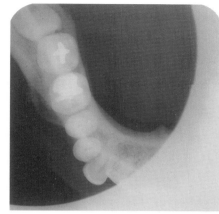

Fig. 8.27 F 28

Films: panoramic, periapical, and lower true occlusal.

There is an oval radiolucent lesion in the right body of the mandible surrounding mesial root of 46, extending from distal of 45 to distal root of 46, and from 2 mm below alveolar crest to upper border of ID canal. Clearly radiolucent on the panoramic film, there is a graininess to the content of the lesion on the periapical; the margins are well defined and corticated; 46 is heavily restored and there is probability of pulpal involvement; the occlusal view shows buccal expansion with thinning of the overlying cortical bone. Although the lesion extends to the root of 45 the cortical outline of the socket is still intact.

Impression: a benign, expansile lesion, possibly containing more than one tissue type (the graininess), which may be odontogenic in origin.

Differential diagnosis: cemento-ossifying lesion; radicular cyst; solitary bone cyst; odontogenic keratocyst.

Follow-up: the tooth was removed and the lesion enucleated; the histology indicated a fibro-osseous lesion; in view of its relation to the tooth it was unclear as to whether it should be labelled periapical cemental dysplasia or cemento-ossifying fibroma.

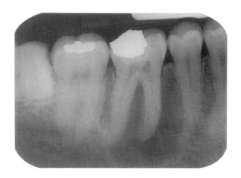

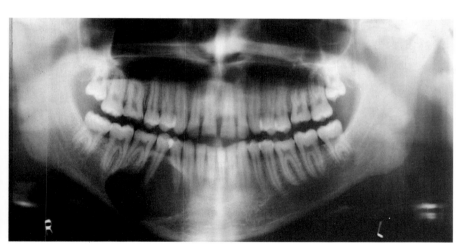

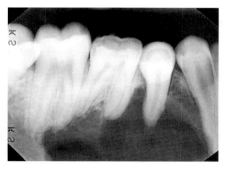

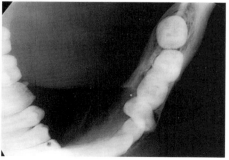

Fig. 8.28 M 20, self-referred complaining of non-painful swelling right body of mandible, slowly expanding.

Films: panoramic, periapical, and lower true occlusal.

There is a loculated extensive radiolucency in the right body of the mandible, extending from 43 to 47, and from just below the crest of the ridge to the lower border of the mandible; the margins are well defined but not corticated; the teeth show evidence of displacement: all are unrestored but 46 shows evidence of chronological hypoplasia occlusally; there is marked buccal and lingual expansion with thinning of the overlying cortex.

Impression: a benign but rapidly expansile lesion, probably not cystic (lack of cortication, and not infected: no symptoms), possibly odontogenic in origin.

Differential diagnosis: ameloblastoma; giant cell granuloma; myxoma.

Follow-up: the lesion was biopsied and diagnosed histologically as a central giant cell granuloma; there was no underlying hyperparathyroidism.

Fig. 8.29 F 74, requiring extraction of few remaining teeth, and provision of dentures.
Film: panoramic radiograph.
There is a radiolucent lesion situated near the right angle of the mandible; oval with well-defined and radiopaque margins; 1 cm diameter; it is situated close to the angle of the mandible, below the ID canal, remote from dental structures; there is no effect on other structures.
Impression: a benign 'cystic' lesion, non-odontogenic in origin due to its position below the ID canal.
Provisional diagnosis: Stafne's idiopathic bone cavity. In this situation, where the appearance and site of the lesion match the classic description of a Stafne's idiopathic bone cavity, provided there are no signs or symptoms to indicate further active investigation, the best course of action is to review in 6 or 12 months in order to determine radiologically that there has been no change.

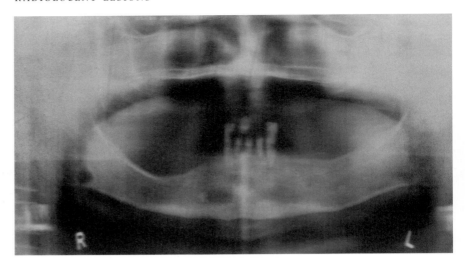

9 Radiopaque and combination lesions

9.1   INTRODUCTION   160
9.2   SITES AND MATERIALS INVOLVED   160
9.3   RADIOPAQUE AND COMBINATION LESIONS   160
    9.3.1 Normal   **164**
    9.3.2 Developmental   **164**
    9.3.3 Inflammatory   **165**
    9.3.4 Cystic   **166**
    9.3.5 Neoplastic   **166**
    9.3.6 Osteodystrophies   **167**
    9.3.7 Metabolic   **167**
    9.3.8 Idiopathic   **167**
    9.3.9 Iatrogenic   **173**
    9.3.10 Foreign bodies   **173**
    9.3.11 Artefacts   **173**

9 Radiopaque and combination lesions

9.1 INTRODUCTION

Any structure that attenuates the X-ray beam sufficiently to prevent photons from reaching the X-ray film or other recording medium, results in radiopaque or white areas within the image. This has been referred to in earlier chapters (Chapters 1 and 2), and is related to the atomic number of the material involved, quantity of the material in the path of the X-ray beam, and the exposure factors.

Many normal structures are relatively radiopaque, notably the dental hard tissues and cortical bone. This chapter is primarily concerned with radiographic features presumed to be caused by abnormalities, and analysis of the descriptive appearance, in order to determine the cause of the variation. Images exhibiting a degree of radiolucency as well as radiopacity have been included as it is their radiopaque component that frequently alerts the observer to their presence; this group includes situations where it is predominantly the pattern of a feature that is perceived to have been altered.

9.2 SITES AND MATERIALS INVOLVED

All sites included in the field of view of a radiographic image will be demonstrable if they incorporate some feature that sufficiently attenuates the X-ray beam to result in a radiopaque image. This is quite different to radiolucencies that are only perceived due to their contrast with surrounding radiopaque images; they can usually be identified as being within bone, or within a tooth. Radiopacities may also be within bone, or teeth, but there is as much chance of them being within adjacent soft tissues. Examples of the various mechanisms for creating radiopacities are given in Chapter 3. Most radiographic images contain a number of different known materials, which can be used to match the unknown lesion, in order to determine the likely tissue type, or other material from which it is constructed.

It is important to identify the location of a radiopacity accurately, as an initial step in determining the possible material or tissue involved. Radiographic localization methods (Chapter 4) can be applied, to supplement a thorough clinical examination.

9.3 RADIOPAQUE AND COMBINATION LESIONS

The examples used in this chapter will illustrate the value of the descriptive features of a lesion. The categories of the radiological sieve will provide the framework, and a list of lesions that fall within each category will be provided, although not all will be illustrated.

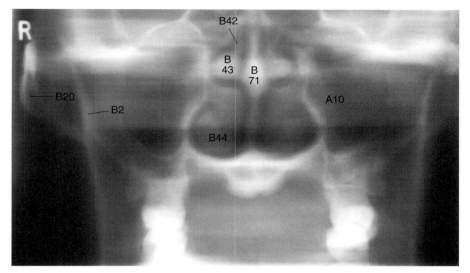

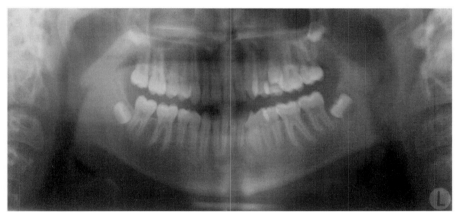

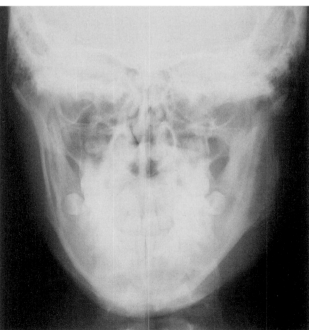

Fig. 9.1 F 32, presenting with a bony hard symmetrical swelling in the hard palate; no symptoms; duration of swelling unknown.

Film: coronal tomogram through the centre of the lesion, and the molar teeth.

There is a very radiopaque bilobed structure extending approximately 1 cm to either side of the midline of the palate; the degree of opacity matches the crowns of the teeth; the margins are clearly demarcated, and there are bilateral radiolucencies related to the palatal surface between the lesion and the floor of the nasal cavity, which is unaltered.

Impression: the lesion cannot be constructed of enamel as there is no recognizable tooth form; the high degree of opacity is therefore suggestive of cortical bone. This is a common site for developmental exostoses.

Provisional diagnosis: torus palatinus.

The clinical and radiological appearance are both typical of torus palatinus and no further investigations are indicated. Treatment (removal) is only necessary if the lesion interferes with denture retention.

The anatomical codes conform with the lists in Appendix B.

Fig. 9.2 M 15, presented complaining of increasing size of left lower jaw, non-painful, occurring over a number of weeks.

Films: panoramic and PA mandible.

There is an increase in size of the whole height of the left ramus, antero-posteriorly and laterally, expanding the outline of the mandible, except laterally where the original lateral margin can still be seen within the altered ramus; the pattern of the bone is finer than that of the body region; there is no margin delineating the altered bone; the developing 38 is related to the area and has an enlarged follicular space, which is not fully covered by bone; the ID canal is not clearly seen on either side.

Impression: a pathological lesion causing an alteration in the nature and size of the left ramus of the mandible; the marked increase in size over a relatively short period of time is suggestive of neoplastic change until proven otherwise.

Differential diagnosis: osteosarcoma; fibrous dysplasia; osteomyelitis.

Follow-up: the bone was biopsied distobuccal to 38, and a CT examination was carried out (see Appendix D, Fig. D9); the biopsy provided a diagnosis of osteomyelitis. The cause is unclear as there is no related dental pathology, except for the enlarged 38 follicle, which may be causative, or the result of the infection.

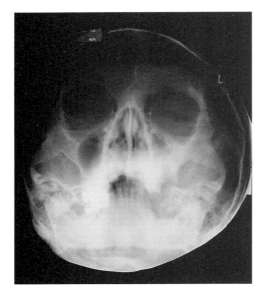

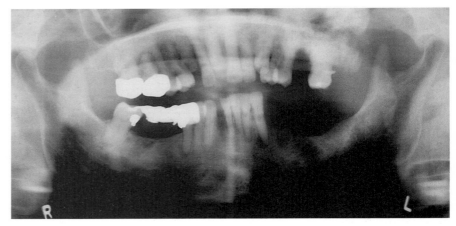

Fig. 9.3 M 78, 1-year history of pain and swelling in left maxilla, treated with antibiotics; swelling and draining sinuses both buccally and palatally.

Films: panoramic and OM view, taken after extraction of 27.

Partially edentulous, heavily restored dentition, with missing 26 (recently extracted); the left posterior maxilla is relatively more radiopaque than on the right, the affected area blending into normal bone in the premolar region; the increase in opacity is not uniform, and the areas are of irregular shapes; the OM view shows marked thickening of the lateral wall of the left maxilla, and opacification of the lower part of the sinus.

Impression: the radiological appearance on the OM view could be the result of malignancy or inflammatory change; the history and clinical findings are valuable in the differentiation; the panoramic appearance is more suggestive of
non-uniform inflammatory change.

Differential diagnosis: chronic diffuse sclerosing osteomyelitis (CDSO); infected neoplasm.

Follow-up: the lesion was biopsied, confirming a diagnosis of CDSO, which was treated by debridement and a long course of antibiotic therapy.

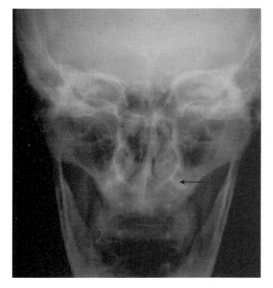

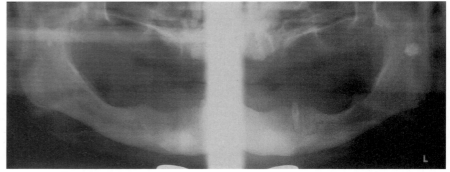

Fig. 9.4a M 64, requiring full dentures; panoramic radiograph taken to check for roots in addition to clinically evident 32.

Films: panoramic and PA Mandible (taken as a view at right-angles).

On the panoramic film there is a very radiopaque, 1 cm diameter, circular mass in the region of the left lingula, with a non-uniform consistency and a clear margin. The PA view demonstrates that it is lingual to the mandible and must therefore be within soft tissue; there is a similar, smaller, opacity on the right.

Impression: it is very unusual to see variations in the degree of mineralization of the ramus of the mandible; the opacity is greater than that of any normal structure within the image indicating a very dense material or substantial thickness; the site is typical for superimposition of tonsillar calcifications, and the correct position is confirmed by the PA view (arrowed).

Diagnosis: tonsillar calcification related to recurrent infective episodes.

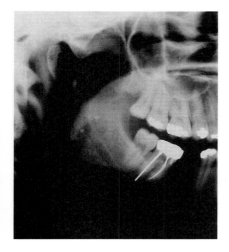
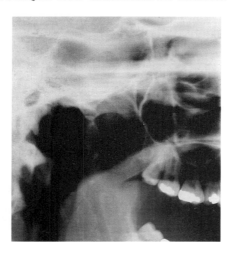

Fig. 9.4b F 35, tonsillar calcifications detected as a chance finding on open and closed panoramic views taken for TMJs (temporo-mandibular joints): note how the small radiopacities have altered their positional relationship with the ramus.

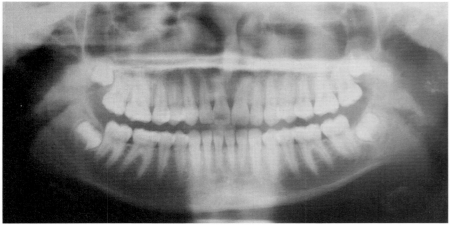

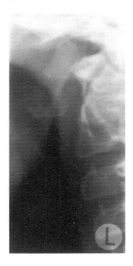

Fig. 9.5 F 14, radiographic assessment for orthodontic treatment.

Films: panoramic radiograph, PA mandible, sectional panoramic (all different dates).
On comparing the right and left sides of the panoramic image an area of discrete small radiopacities is evident in the region of the left ramus, level with the lingula, and extending distal to the ramus; the overall shape is almost circular, 1.5 cm diameter but there is no external margin. The PA view was taken as a view at right-angles, and to give a clearer image of the radiopaque mass which is clearly within the buccal soft tissues; the sectional panoramic view was taken 8 months later and shows no change in the quantity or degree of the opaque lesion (other than attributable to technique).

Impression: the original image is suggestive of soft tissue calcification, and a thorough clinical examination was carried out which revealed a firm, mobile mass within the left cheek; no symptoms; duration of mass unknown; history of lengthy bout of mumps affecting left parotid gland.

Provisional diagnosis: in view of the position, the medical history, and the radiological appearance, which is strongly suggestive of inflammatory deposition of calcium in soft tissues, a provisional diagnosis of parotid calcification can be made; sialography would assist in substantiating this but was not indicated in view of the lack of symptoms.

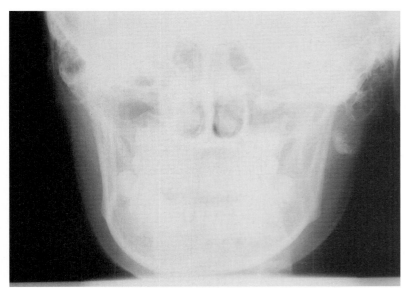

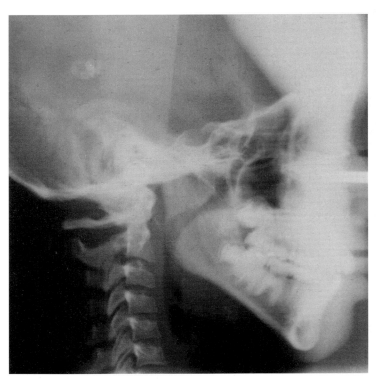 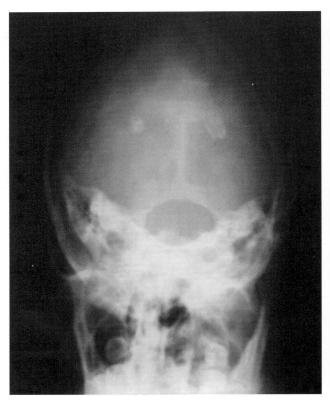

Fig. 9.6   F 13, radiographic examination as part of orthodontic evaluation.
Films: lateral ceph., Reverse Towne's.
There is an unusual irregular shaped area of non-uniform opacity above and behind the image of the ear in the lateral ceph. The Reverse Towne's view was taken as a view almost at right-angles to determine the location and demonstrates bilateral, symmetrical, circular areas of opacity; approximately 1.5 cm diameter with clearly defined margins; not radiologically related to any other feature.
Impression: the symmetrical, non-uniform radiopacities are chance findings on routine radiographs, and have an appearance similar to other soft tissue calcifications. Their site in relation to the midline, and vertical and antero-posterior position are indicative of calcified choroid plexus.
Provisional diagnosis: calcified choroid plexus of unknown origin.
This condition can occur in relation to infection with cytomegalovirus, cat-scratch fever, and for no known cause. No treatment is indicated unless an underlying condition is detected.

Each example of a radiopacity or combination lesion will use the common list of significant features, to provide a description that aids their comparison. The *impression* that is given by the combination of features will be discussed, and the provisional or differential diagnosis provided, together with the follow up and actual diagnosis where this is relevant. The lesions which are illustrated are marked with an asterisk (*) in the lists that follow; a number of the lesions are illustrated elsewhere.

9.3.1   Normal

● Teeth
● Bones

9.3.2   Developmental

● Extra Cusps
● Supernumerary teeth

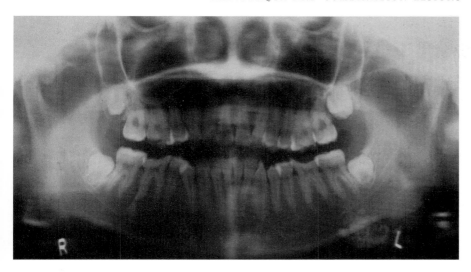

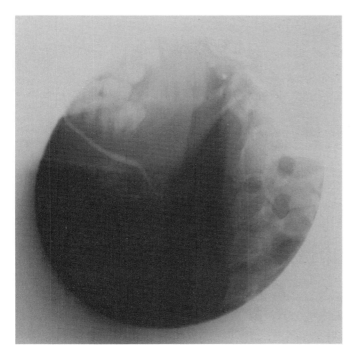

Fig. 9.7 F 17, attending for first dental examination, no symptoms.
(a) *Film*: panoramic.
The dentition is not complete with missing 15 and 22; there is wearing down of the occlusal surfaces of the first molars, and lower central incisors, and clinically enamel irregularities affecting the upper central incisors and canines. The most notable feature is a collection of radiopacities forming a near circle, 1.5 cm diameter, superimposed on the lower border of the left mandible; the normal bony architecture can be seen through the lesion.

There was a firm, moveable mass palpable infero-lingual to the lower border of the mandible.

Impression: a dental developmental abnormality and a soft tissue calcification of inflammatory origin.

Differential diagnosis: chronological hypoplasia affecting incisors, canines, and first molars; calcified submandibular salivary gland; calcified lymph node.
(b) *Film*: left submandibular sialogram.
There is incomplete filling of the ductal system within the left submandibular salivary gland; in spite of this the main duct can be seen to pass by the opaque mass which is quite separate.
Diagnosis: calcified lymph node. Although there was very little accurate information about the medical history, it is possible that the same illness that is implicated in the dental hypoplasia is implicated in the lymph node; the patient spent her infanthood in mainland China in an area where tuberculosis is widespread.

- Odontomes
- Exostosis: torus palatinus*, torus mandibularis

9.3.3 Inflammatory

- Sclerosing osteitis
- Chronic (sclerosing) osteomyelitis*
- Sequestra
- Callus formation secondary to fracture
- Hypercementosis
- Calcified lymph nodes, and other lymphatic tissue*
- Sialoliths

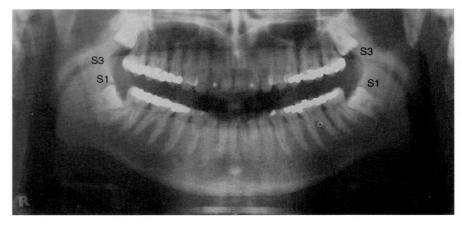

Fig. 9.8   M 20, radiographic examination for orthodontic assessment.
Film: panoramic.
Well-restored dentition including cingulum pit amalgams in 12 and 22; 38 and 48 are
mesio-angular impacted and have not completed root formation; in the right maxillary sinus
there are two domed radiopacities partially superimposed on each other, having a similar opacity
to the soft tissue images of the tongue and soft palate (labelled); approximately 1.5 cm diameter,
they appear to arise from the floor of the sinus; clear superior free margins.
   Impression: any feature within the maxillary sinus other than the normal air appears relatively
radiopaque; these two lesions appear to be benign, expansile, and provably cystic.
   Differential diagnosis: mucous retention cysts; radicular cysts; keratocysts; carcinomas.
   As there are two virtually identical lesions it is extremely unlikely that they are due to
malignant change, particularly in such a young patient; the relationship of the lesions to the
dentition does not favour odontogenic lesions, although the teeth should be examined and the
patient questioned about symptoms. In the absence of any positive findings these lesions can be
diagnosed as mucous retention cysts, single ones being a not infrequent finding on panoramic
radiographs.

- Other soft tissue 'stones', including phleboliths, antroliths, rhinoliths
- Acne scars

9.3.4   Cystic

- Cystic lesions within the antrum
  - radicular
  - dentigerous*
  - keratocyst
  - mucous retention*
- Calcifying epithelial odontogenic cyst (see Fig. 8.16)

9.3.5   Neoplastic

- Benign:
  - ossifying/cementifying fibroma*
  - cementoma
  - cementoblastoma*
  - osteoma*
  - calcifying epithelial odontogenic tumour

- Malignant:
  - osteogenic sarcoma*

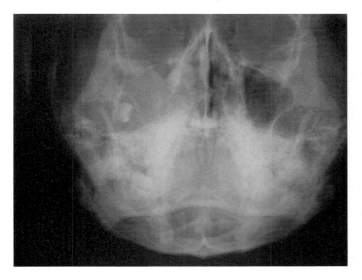
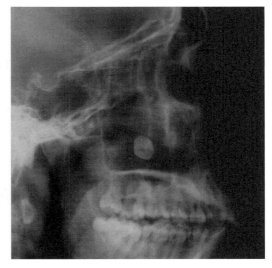
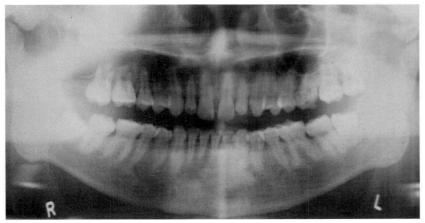
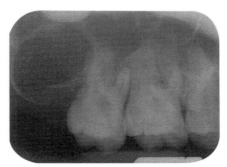

Fig. 9.9   M 24, complaining of swelling of right maxilla, otherwise asymptomatic.
Films: panoramic, periapical, OM, lateral facial bones.
The right maxillary sinus is almost completely obliterated by a lesion that is radiolucent on the intra-oral and lateral views and radiopaque on the others; associated with the crown of an ectopic, developing third molar, seen lateral to the normal lateral margin of the sinus on the OM, with its occlusal surface facing into the lesion, which appears to be attached to its neck. The vertical position of the tooth varies between the different lateral projections due to its position buccal to the arch.

   Impression: a benign, cystic lesion involving the developing upper right third molar, present for some considerable time.

   Differential diagnosis: dentigerous cyst (18); keratocyst.

   Follow-up: aspiration biopsy is useful to determine which of these two lesions is the correct diagnosis on the basis of the soluble protein content (lower in keratocysts than other cystic lesions).

9.3.6   Osteodystrophies

- Fibrous dysplasia*
- Cherubism

9.3.7   Metabolic

- Paget's disease of bone*
- Hyperparathyroidism

9.3.8   Idiopathic

- Osteosclerosis*

Fig. 9.10 M 43, complaining of recent difficulty in chewing related to slowly enlarging mass attached to left maxillary alveolus, and present for a number of years.
Films: bitewing and periapical.
A pedunculated, smooth outlined, bony mass is attached to the left maxillary alveolar ridge in the region where the molars are no longer present; covered by a thin cortical layer, the bulk shows a fine trabecular pattern continuous with that of the alveolus; the periapical has been taken with the film buccal to the lower teeth which are overlapped with the lesion in the bitewing.

   Impression: a benign, bony growth.

   Provisional diagnosis: osteoma (exostosis).

   Follow-up: the lesion was removed at the level of the alveolus, for functional reasons; the diagnosis was confirmed.

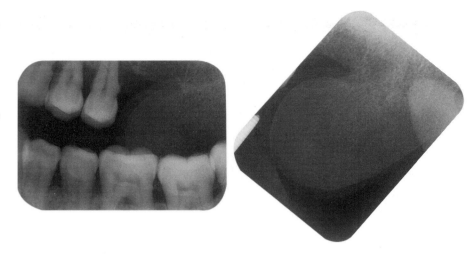

Fig. 9.11 F 29, referred for investigation of asymptomatic, hard, expansile lesion in left mandible.
Films: panoramic and lower true occlusal. (See also Figs 3.15 and 3.29.)
There is a spherical radiopaque lesion in the left body of the mandible, related to the apex of 35, surrounded by a narrow radiolucent zone; the lesion is approximately 2 cm in diameter and is of non-uniform radiopacity; in the panoramic radiograph it is more radiopaque than bony structures, but almost identical in the occlusal view: this is the truer indication of its possible tissue type; the apex of 35 is masked by the lesion; the ID canal is not altered; the cortical bone at the adjacent lower border of the mandible is thickened, whereas the lingual and buccal cortical plates have been destroyed.
Impression: a benign, slow-growing tumour containing mineralized tissue (bone or cementum), causing a low-grade inflammatory response in parts of the adjacent bone.
Differential diagnosis: cementoblastoma; ossifying/cementifying fibroma; complex odontome. The lesion as seen on the panoramic radiograph is opaque enough to contain enamel, but not on the occlusal view; ossifying/cementifying fibromas are not normally surrounded by a radiolucent zone; the appearance is typical of a cementoblastoma, which was proven histologically after enucleation.

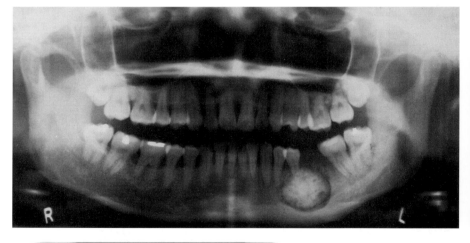

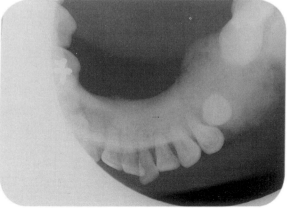

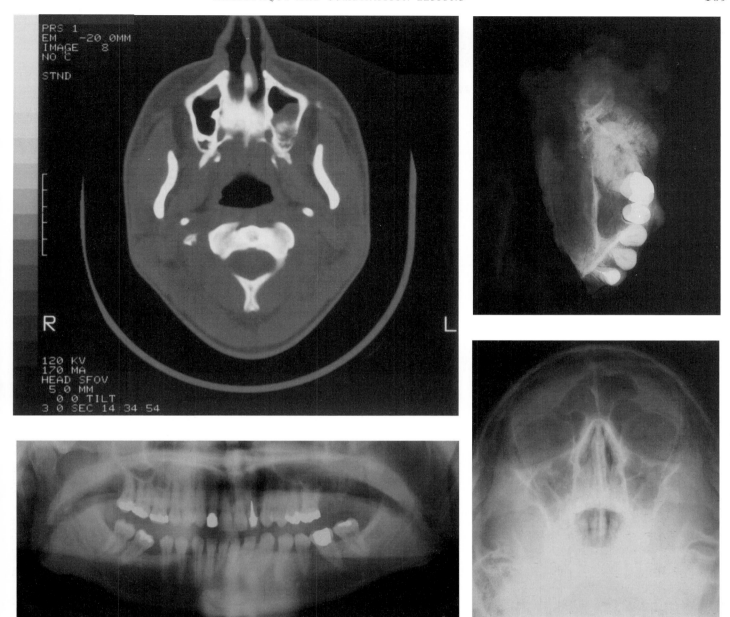

Fig. 9.12   M 26, complaining of painless swelling in left upper buccal sulcus of fairly short duration, referred by dentist after extraction of 27 and antibiotic therapy failed to resolve the swelling.

Films: panoramic, OM, CT scan.

Periapicals and an oblique occlusal were not very helpful in this case.

The outline of the left maxillary sinus has been lost on the panoramic view distal to 26; the alveolus in the region of 27/28 shows a subtle change in pattern compared to the contralateral side; on the OM view there is evidence of a soft tissue or cystic swelling in the lower part of the maxillary sinus with a fairly flat upper surface.

Impression: at this stage in the patient's investigation the radiographs were not particularly helpful, but in view of the short history, and the lack of any response to antibiotics, it was decided to investigate the possibility of malignancy and CT scans were arranged.

On the axial CT scans taken 2 weeks later there is clear evidence of mineralization within the soft tissue mass in the left maxillary sinus, combined with destruction of the bony margins and the alveolus.

Provisional diagnosis: osteogenic osteosarcoma.

Follow-up: biopsy was arranged to be followed without delay by definitive surgery. The biopsy confirmed the diagnosis and a partial maxillectomy was carried out.

The radiograph of the specimen shows the striking appearance of rapid bone formation within the lesion.

Fig. 9.13 F 47, self-referred requesting provision of dentures, no symptoms, aware of asymmetry between right and left sides of the upper jaw.
Film: panoramic.
There is an obvious increase in size of the right maxillary alveolus distal to 13, clinically evident buccally and palatally; the bone has an even finer pattern than the equivalent area on the left, this pattern blending almost imperceptibly with the normal bone supporting the anterior teeth; there is no definable margin to the affected area; the overlying soft tissue is of normal thickness.

   Impression: a non-developmental, non-inflammatory, non-malignant lesion causing an increase in size and alteration of the internal structure of the right maxilla, of unknown duration.

   Provisional diagnosis: fibrous dysplasia: the altered appearance is typical of fibrous dysplasia which causes a *ground-glass* appearance, which typically blends with the adjacent bone.

   Follow-up: biopsy can be used to confirm the diagnosis. Treatment is aimed at reduction of size in order to improve functional and aesthetic characteristics, if required.

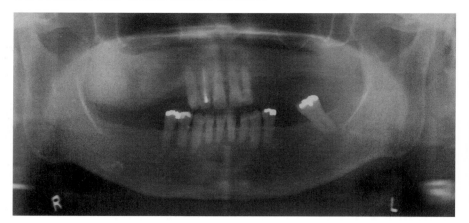

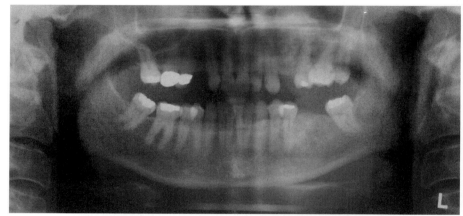

Fig. 9.14   (centre figure, and right) F 40, referred by general practitioner for investigation of unusual appearance of bone detected on bitewing radiographs; no symptoms.
Films: panoramic and OM.
There are two areas of altered appearance on the panoramic radiograph related to the partially edentulous upper left premolar and lower left molar regions. Both show whorls of radiopacity alternating with radiolucent patches, within an area of approximately 2 cm diameter; the margins of the lower lesion are not clearly defined, but those of the upper lesion can be detected, particularly the upper margin within the maxillary sinus seen on both views; the related teeth are not affected.

   Impression: two areas of altered bone, both in sites where teeth are missing, and there is therefore a possibility of inflammatory origin.

   Differential diagnosis: chronic sclerosing osteomyelitis; ossifying/cementifying fibroma; fibrous dysplasia.

   Follow-up: the lower lesion was biopsied, resulting in a histological diagnosis of a fibro-osseous lesion. The patient did not wish surgical intervention and radiological follow-up was instituted.

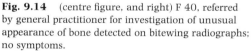

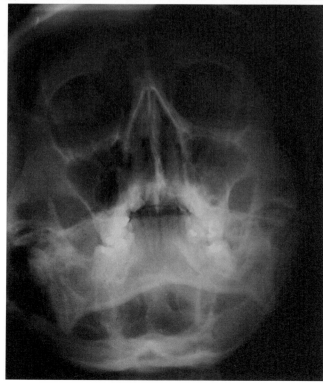

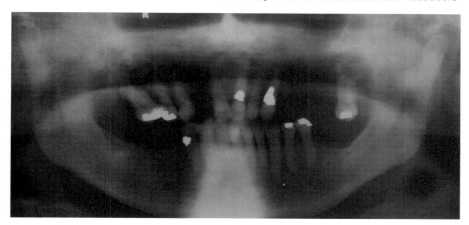

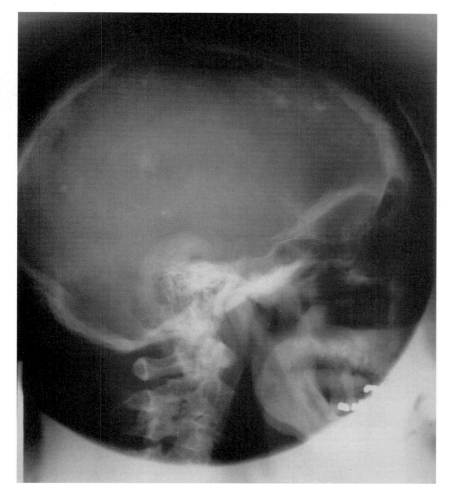

Fig 9.15 M 61, requiring new partial dentures due to difficulty in wearing present set.
Films: panoramic and lateral skull view.
The trabecular pattern of the mandible is normal; in contrast there are multiple patches of radiopacity in both right and left maxillae, predominantly in the molar regions; patchy irregular shaped radiopacities can also be seen in the skull vault, which is itself thicker than normal; the increase in opacity of the maxilla is very clear in the lateral view; there is a suggestion of hypercementosis affecting 17, 15, 27, and 35; generalized horizontal bone loss.

Impression: the extensive alteration of bone pattern in a late-middle-aged patient is indicative of a widespread alteration of the normal physiology of bone turnover, as seen in Paget's disease.

Provisional diagnosis: Paget's disease of bone.

Follow-up: the diagnosis can be confirmed by a raised serum alkaline phosphatase level, and increased urinary calcium and hydroxyproline levels. There is no treatment for Paget's disease; symptomatic treatment may be required for the neurological symptoms that can follow, related to the pattern of bone deposition.

Fig. 9.16   F 16, examination related to dental crowding, and to investigate presence of third molars. *Film*: panoramic.

There is a tear-drop shaped uniformly radiopaque area between the roots of the lower right canine and premolar, extending from the alveolar crest to 2 mm above the cortical lower border of the mandible, from mesial to the root of the premolar and the mental foramen, to mesial to the root of the canine; the other premolar has been previously extracted; the margin is clearly delineated, and blends with the lamina dura of the involved teeth; the teeth are sound ,as are all the teeth with the exception of restored 26 and 36; the third molars are developing in good positions; the central incisors are shovel shaped and 21 may be invaginated (the patient is of Asian origin); the earrings have not been removed and their ghost images can be seen just below the orbital margins.

Impression: an area of highly sclerotic bone related to two teeth close to the site of a missing tooth, inflammatory or idiopathic in origin.

Differential diagnosis: idiopathic osteosclerosis; sclerosing osteitis.

Follow-up: the related teeth tested vital, supporting the first diagnosis. Although the affected bone may originally have arisen in relation to the missing tooth, the extraction was related to crowding and not dental pathology; radiological review in a year is recommended to ensure there is no change.

The body of the mandible is a common site for areas of increased mineralization for no clear reason.

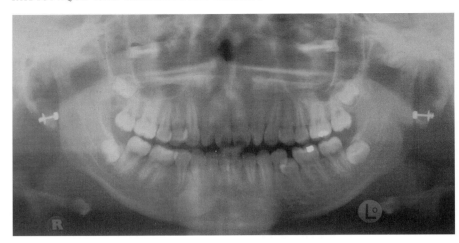

Fig. 9.17   F 53
Film: panoramic.

In addition to the radiopaque restorations related to most of the upper teeth there is an irregular shaped radiopaque (metal) area above and remote from the apex of 21(a); the mesial portion is rod-like; the distal portion resembles half a clam shell with the serrations distally; its greatest length is approximately 1 cm; well-defined margins; the soft tissue image of the nose can be seen extending from 13 to 23 and related to the object.

Impression: a foreign body present in the alveolus, nasal cavity, or soft tissue of the nose: because of the width of the plane in focus anteriorly it is unlikely to be outside the patient and still depicted so clearly.

Diagnosis: clinical examination revealed a nose ring that had not been removed prior to radiography. Removable objects should be removed as they may be superimposed on areas of interest and reduce the radiological value of the image.

Radiolucent markes (b) are due to pressure artefacts.

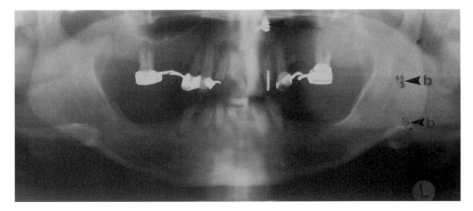

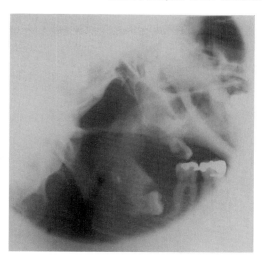

Fig. 9.18   M 54
Film: oblique lateral of right ramus.
There is a small radiopaque angular area above the upper border of the ID canal near to the lingula region; similar radiopacity to metal restorations; approximately 2 mm wide × 3 mm high, with well-defined margins.

   Impression: metal foreign body in patient, or outside patient in path of beam, or foreign body in cassette: there is a need to check the cassette; examine the patient's clothing, check the history — in order depending on outcome.

   Follow-up, and diagnosis: on examination of the cassette there was a piece of paper on one of the intensifying screens which will have been sufficient to prevent the emitted light from reaching the film: no light results in no sensitization of the emulsion, and therefore a white patch, as occurs when metal attenuates the beam.

   Note also the increased size of the follicle associated with 48 (see Fig. 8.5.).

9.3.9   Iatrogenic

- Restorations
- Amalgam tattoos
- Endodontic instruments
- Surgical treatment accessories (e.g. plates, wires, staples)

9.3.10   Foreign bodies

- Metal fragments of various sorts*
- Some fish or animal bone fragments

9.3.11   Artefacts

- dust on intensifying screens*

Information concerning the pathology of the lesions listed and illustrated, can be found in standard texts and those listed in the Bibliography.

10 Dental trauma

10.1 INTRODUCTION   176
10.2 CAUSES OF DENTAL TRAUMA   176
    10.2.1 Acute   **176**
    10.2.2 Chronic   **181**
10.3 RADIOGRAPHY   182
    10.3.1 The acute physically assaulted tooth **182**
    10.3.2 The non-physically assaulted tooth   **183**
10.4 RADIOLOGICAL APPEARANCE   183

10   Dental trauma

10.1   INTRODUCTION

The face and dentition are relatively unprotected parts of the human body. Although the soft tissues of the face provide some protection to the posterior teeth, the anterior dentition is frequently exposed. Traumatic injury can be caused by a variety of factors; some are obvious, such as physical violence, others can cause as much damage but are less obvious, such as chronic chemical trauma from personal habits (e.g. excessive fizzy drink consumption).

This chapter will classify the types of trauma to which teeth are prone, discuss the place of radiography in the examination, and illustrate a selection of the variety of radiological appearances.

Trauma affecting the alveolar bone and the basal portions of the mandible and maxillae will not be discussed. They are well covered in other texts, and their treatment is normally outside the remit of the general dental practitioner.

10.2   CAUSES OF DENTAL TRAUMA

Trauma to the dentition can be classified in a number of ways: acute or chronic; physical or chemical; self-inflicted or resulting from external forces; intentional or accidental. There is considerable cross-over between such groups, and an attempt will be made here to collate the most important divisions under two major headings: acute and chronic. In each of these groups there is inclusion of important, but avoidable, iatrogenic causes of traumatic damage to dental tissues.

10.2.1   Acute

Physical

Direct physical injury
Intentional or unintentional;
visible or invisible damage.

Results in:
● Fracture: crown
— through enamel only, enamel and dentine, or enamel, dentine and pulp (Fig. 10.1);
— horizontal, vertical, oblique.

Fractures of the crown of the tooth are evident on clinical examination, which will reveal which of the dental tissues are involved. The pulp is at risk when the fracture runs through dentine, as well as when there is frank pulpal expo-

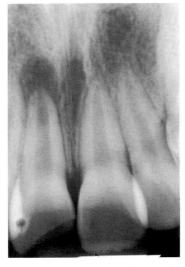

Fig. 10.1   Mesial fracture through enamel and dentine of 11, resulting in periapical inflammation: F 9.

sure, due to the communication that is opened up through the dentinal tubules. If there is associated soft tissue injury then the examination should investigate the possibility of tooth fragments, or other foreign material, being within the soft tissue.

- Fracture: root
    — and crown, or root alone (Figs 10.2–10.8);
    — horizontal, vertical, oblique;
    — coronal, middle, or apical third.

- Avulsion, normally of whole tooth (Figs 10.9 and 10.10) most commonly affects single-rooted teeth. It is important to determine where the tooth is as it may be possible to reimplant it. In situations where there has been loss of consciousness, even momentarily, there is a possibility that the tooth, or a broken fragment, has been inhaled, and this requires investigation (Fig. 10.11).

- Subluxation, or displacement of tooth (Figs 10.12–10.14).

- Damage to the apical blood vessels, with or without physical damage, can result in a loss of vitality which may only be detected at a much later date

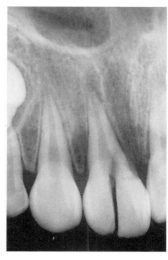

Fig. 10.2 Vertical fracture through the crown and coronal root of 11; removal of the separated fragment is necessary and restorative treatment of the remaining portion will be complicated by the level of the fracture. There is already a clear area of periapical inflammatory change secondary to pulp death: F 10.

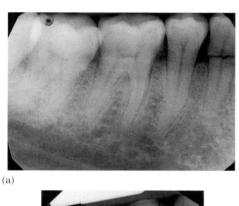

(a)

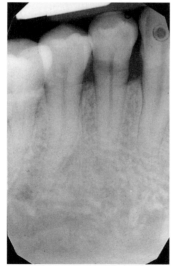

(b)

Fig. 10.3
(a) Clear horizontal fracture through coronal root of 44: M 44.
(b) Bisecting angle periapical causing overlap of the fragments, mimicking cervical radiolucency.

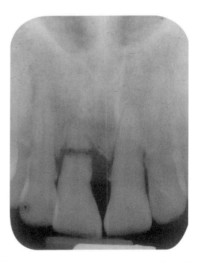

Fig. 10.4 Masticatory injury to periodontally involved 11; calculus on proximal surfaces, and vertical bone loss: M 56.

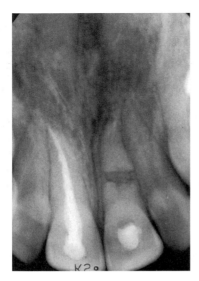

due to discoloration of the crown, or a chance finding on a radiograph (Fig. 10.15).

Iatrogenic: non-intentional, related to dental treatment.
Excessive heat during cavity preparation, or amalgam polishing; pulpal exposure.

Results in:
- Acute inflammatory changes in the pulpal tissue, which will progress to pulpal death if appropriate action is not immediately taken.

Fig. 10.5 Horizontal mid-third root fracture; 22 months after injury there is evidence of a bone bridge between the fragments: M 13.

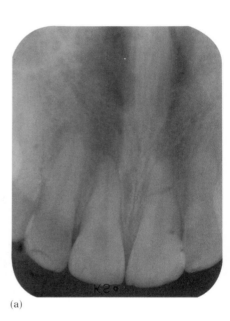

(a)

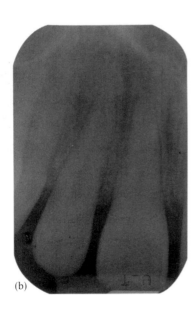

(b)

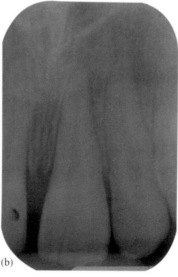

(b)

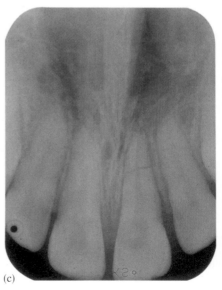

(c)

Fig. 10.6
(a) Horizontal root fracture through apical portion of root of 21; minimal separation of fragments. The widening of the distal periodontal ligament space indicates a degree of subluxation of the tooth: M 13.
(b) 5 months later the periapicals fail to show the fracture, although there is evidence of periapical inflammatory change related to 21; these periapicals have been taken using the paralleling technique (evidence of film holders) and the vertical beam angulation is therefore similar to that used in panoramic radiography.
Bisecting angle periapical (to match original film) 1 week later showed the fracture unchanged as does this film (c) taken 9 months later; there has been no further separation of the two fragments in spite of active removable orthodontic treatment.
The appearance of the fracture in the bisecting angle films and not in the paralleling films indicates that this fracture line is oblique, running from a more inferior level on the palatal aspect to a more superior level on the buccal aspect.

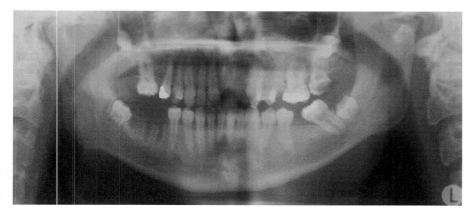

Fig. 10.9   21 has been completely avulsed as a result of direct trauma, and not re-implanted; note the clear radiopaque outline of the socket: although the injury occurred 3 weeks previously remodelling has not commenced: M 17.

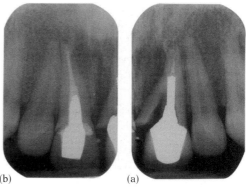

Fig. 10.7
(a) Oblique fracture through root of 21, related to post-crown: M 36.
(b) Parallax periapical determines the relative buccal position of the free edge of the fragment.

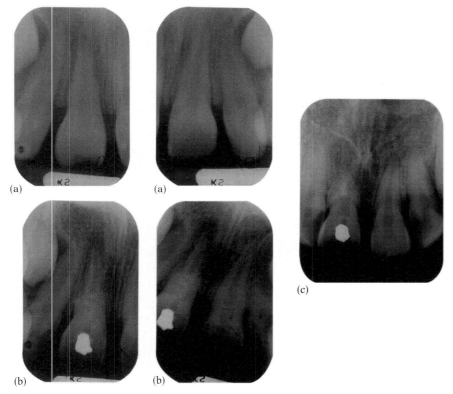

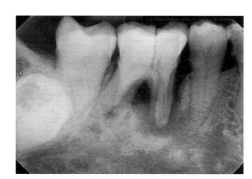

Fig. 10.8   Vertical fracture through periodontally compromised 46: F 76.

Fig. 10.10
(a) 11 has been avulsed and re-implanted; there is loss of definition of the socket outline, evidence of inflammatory bone change, and root resorption affecting the apex and mesial surface of the root: F 20.
(b) 8 months later after treatment with calcium hydroxide there is still evidence of root resorption.
(c) 38 months after the injury the root is severely reduced in length; an apical fragment still persists.

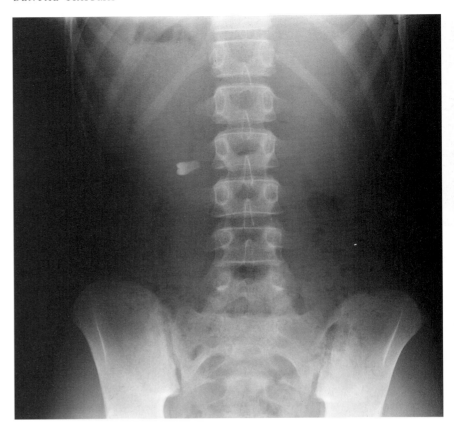

Fig. 10.11   A premolar tooth that has been swallowed, rather than inhaled: F 11.

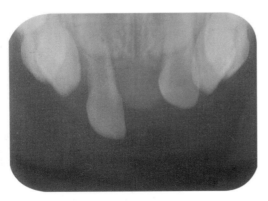

Fig. 10.12   Displacement of 61 (upper left deciduous central incisor) due to direct trauma 1 week previously; radiography at this stage is worthwhile to demonstrate any change in position of the permanent successor: M 2.

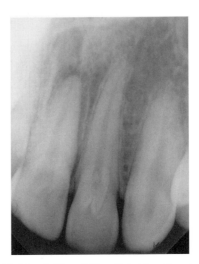

Fig. 10.13   Subluxed 21 with 'widened' periodontal ligament space; 22 is invaginated: M 11.

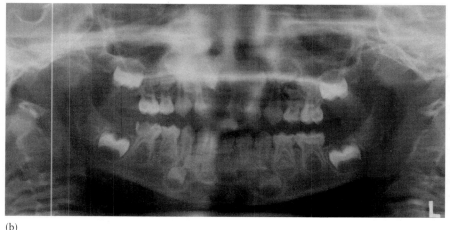
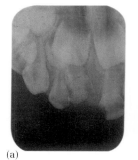
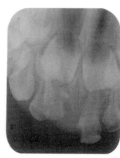

(b)

(a)

Fig. 10.14
(a) Buccally displaced 51 appearing only slightly intruded on these bisecting angle periapicals: M 4.
(b) On the panoramic film the tooth is barely visible due to parallax displacement.

Chemical

Iatrogenic
Application of noxious chemicals to the pulp surface.

10.2.2 Chronic

Physical

Self-inflicted
Attrition; abrasion; habits; excessive chronic occlusal forces. Any attack on a tooth's integrity will initiate a response in the vital pulp, which is demonstrated by secondary dentine deposition; there is a limit to how fast this can be laid down, and there often comes a time when the pulp is unable to protect itself and loss of vitality follows. Prior to this most habitual tooth wear has its own characteristic radiological appearance (Fig. 10.16).

Iatrogenic
Heat transfer through unlined metal restorations; uneven occlusal forces resulting from placement of restorations, or altered occlusion after orthodontic treatment.

Chemical

Self-inflicted
Erosion (Fig. 10.17), resulting from: excessive fizzy drink consumption; habits, such as sucking lemon wedges; acid regurgitation from the stomach; eating disorders, such as bulimia.

Iatrogenic
Micro-leakage in relation to chemical dental dressings and around inadequately packed restorations.

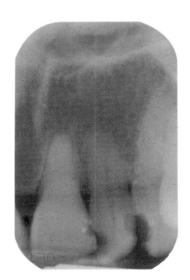

Fig. 10.15 Sclerosed pulp canal in 21 resulting from trauma many years previously; the periapical tissues are normal: F 45.

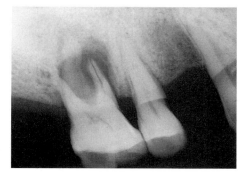

Fig. 10.16 Toothbrush abrasion of 13, 15, and 16; the radiological signs are clearest on the smaller teeth 13 and 15; 16 has become non-vital resulting in periapical rarefying osteitis: M 52.

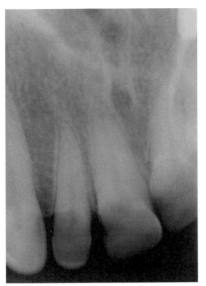

Fig. 10.17   Loss of enamel due to erosion: M 27.

10.3   RADIOGRAPHY

The various types of trauma to the dental tissues result in a variety of immediate and long-term effects. Radiography is not always indicated, for example, iatrogenic exposure of the pulp does not require a radiograph for confirmation, although a radiograph may be indicated as an integral part of any subsequent endodontic treatment.

Teeth which have been physically assaulted require radiographic examination, even if apparently undamaged, in order to detect non-visible damage and provide a base line for future management.

Teeth which have not been physically assaulted may still require planned radiographic examination, which will be indicated by subsequent signs or symptoms relating to the tooth, or a chance finding on an existing radiograph.

These two quite different categories will be dealt with separately in the following sections.

10.3.1   The acute physically assaulted tooth

Radiographic examination is an important part of the examination following obvious acute physical trauma to the teeth. It is essential for positive confirmation of root fractures, and to demonstrate fragments of teeth and foreign bodies in soft tissues. It is important that the radiographs obtained are of good quality and without distortion. The information obtained will have implications in deciding the appropriate treatment and its successful outcome.

Two factors can influence the radiographic examination:

1. *Sensitivity of the patient*: an individual who has suffered trauma to their mouth will be concerned about an examination of the teeth and surrounding structures, and this will influence the choice of technique and the practicalities of carrying out the examination, including the timing.

2. *Radiological demonstration of fracture lines*: the demonstration of a fracture line is dependent on the path of the X-ray beam coinciding with the plane of the fracture; when a fracture is indicated by the clinical examination, but not evident on the radiographs, a further examination needs to be carried out altering the vertical and/or horizontal beam angulation.

The following points can assist in obtaining good quality radiographs of acutely traumatized teeth, and may influence the chosen technique:

1. Awareness of the required information: qualitative or quantitative (e.g. 'Is there a fragment present in the lip?' or 'How far subgingivally does the fracture line extend?'). In the first case, any radiographic projection of the lip will provide the answer, either lateral or straight; in the second an undistorted view of the tooth needs to be obtained.

2. Avoid the necessity to put pressure on traumatized teeth by biting on them, and particularly avoid materials coming into contact with an exposed pulp.

3. Consider using oblique occlusal techniques instead of periapical techniques. Use cotton wool rolls placed between adjacent teeth and the film packet, or bite block, to avoid pressure on damaged teeth.

4. Two views are needed of a tooth suspected of having a root fracture. It is preferable for the patient to have these taken on the same occasion, and the following protocol will be suitable in most cases:

1st radiograph: either a periapical or an oblique occlusal centred on the tooth in question.

2nd radiograph: periapical or oblique occlusal centred on one of the adjacent teeth, preferably with a slightly different vertical angle, in addition to the alteration in horizontal centring point.

If there is a root fracture present it is likely that at least one of the films will demonstrate it; if it is evident on both films then the application of the principle of parallax (Chapter 4) will enable an accurate assessment of the orientation of the fracture line to be made.

In the event that a fracture is present and only evident on one radiograph, it should be possible to plan the required alteration in beam angulation to demonstrate it in a further radiograph.

10.3.2   The non-physically assaulted tooth

Recognition of the effects of trauma is sometimes made years later by an altered appearance of the affected tooth, or the discovery of radiological changes on radiographs taken for some other reason. There is less necessity to have more than one radiograph of a tooth in this situation unless there is doubt as to the radiological findings; if indicated a second radiograph should be taken according to the same guidelines given in the previous section.

10.4   RADIOLOGICAL APPEARANCE

The figures illustrating this chapter have been selected to complement the text and indicate the diverse radiological appearances that may be seen. Situations in which there is no notable radiological finding have not been illustrated.

APPENDIX A
Key components in the dental X-ray tube: checklist

CATHODE AND ANODE

Tungsten: symbol, W; atomic number (Z), 74; melting point, 3410 °C.

1. Production of electrons at cathode: current (7–15 mA) through filament causes a 'boiling-off' of electrons.

2. Target (anode) to interact with electrons to produce X-rays (approx. 1 per cent), as well as heat (approx 99 per cent) and to a small extent other electromagnetic radiations.

Two methods:

(a) continuous (braking) (electron–nucleus) (efficiency related to high atomic number);

(b) characteristic (electron–electron), tungsten characteristic radiation at 58 keV and 68 keV.

ANODE BLOCK

Copper: symbol, Cu; atomic number (Z), 29; melting point, 1080 °C; good conductivity.

Copper is a very good conductor and is important in helping dissipate the tremendous heat created in the tungsten target. It needs a high melting point to withstand the heat.

GLASS ENVELOPE

Glass:
Mainly silica: symbol, Si; atomic number (Z), 14; melting point, 1410 °C.
Glass is relatively transparent to X-rays, but strong enough to contain a vacuum.

LEAD SURROUND

Lead: symbol, Pb; atomic number (Z), 82; melting point, 328 °C.

Lead's high atomic number means it is an efficient absorber of X-rays; surrounds tube except for port exit to prevent leakage radiation.

OIL

Carbon-based compound: symbol, C; atomic number (Z), 6.

1. Insulator (electrical).

2. Conductor of heat.

COLLIMATOR

Lead: collimates X-ray beam to required shape (circular or rectangular), used as a good absorber of X-rays.

FILTERS

Aluminium: symbol, Al; atomic number (Z), 13; melting point, 660 °C.

Remove low energy (useless) X-ray photons. Thickness controlled by law:

   1.5 mm Al ≤ 70 kV.
   2.5 mm Al > 70 kV of which 1.5 mm must be permanent.

Useful atomic numbers (Z)

Aluminium	Al	13
Carbon	C	6
Copper	Cu	29
Lead	Pb	82
Tungsten	W	74
Calcium	Ca	20
bone		12
Soft tissue		7

APPENDIX B
Lists of anatomical features

The lists following are reproduced from Chapter 2. The alphanumeric coding is used to identify anatomical features highlighted throughout the text.

CODING

D = dental structures
B = bones and bony features
J = joints, including sutures
A = air spaces
F = fissures, foramina and depressions
C = canals
S = soft tissues

Some features fall into more than one grouping; they are listed in both groups but have one code, derived from the most appropriate group.

DENTAL STRUCTURES

D1	Enamel
D2	Dentine
D3	Pulp chamber
D4	Cementum
D5	Periodontal ligament space
D6	Lamina dura of tooth socket
D7	Follicle (follicular space)
D8	Tooth germ
D9	Tooth crypt

BONES AND BONY FEATURES

B1	Mandible:	coronoid process	B2
		condylar process	B3
		external oblique ridge	B4
		mylohyoid ridge	B5
		lingula	B6
		ID canal	C7
		mental protuberance	B7
		genial tubercles	B8
		cortical margin	B9

B10	Maxilla:	zygomatic process	B11
		hard palate	B12
		— ghost image	B13
		tuberosity	B14
		inferior margin orbit	B15
		antral septum	B16
		Y-line of Ennis	B17
		canine fossa	B18
B20	Zygoma:	temporal process	B21
B26	Hyoid bone		
B30	Temporal:	squamous	B31
		petrous	B32
		mastoid process	B33
		zygomatic process	B34
		— articular eminence	B35
		glenoid fossa	B36
		styloid process	B37
B40	Nasal:	turbinate bones	B41
		— superior	B42
		— middle	B43
		— inferior	B44
		anterior nasal spine	B45
		nasal septum (vomer)	B71
B50	Frontal		
B51	Parietal		
B52	Occipital		
B53	Sphenoid:	clinoid processes	B54
		— anterior	B55
		— posterior	B56
		sella turcica	B57
		greater wing	B58
		lesser wing	B59
		pterygoid plates	B60
		— lateral	B61
		— medial	B62
		— hamulus	B63
		spine	B64
		innominate line	B65
B70	Ethmoid:	vomer (nasal septum)	B71
		crista galli	B72
B80	cervical spine:	C1 (atlas)	B81
		C2 (axis)	B82

JOINTS, INCLUDING SUTURES

J1	Sagittal suture
J2	Coronal suture
J3	Lambdoid suture

Various sutures between facial bones:

J4	zygomatico-frontal
J5	zygomatico-maxillary
J6	zygomatico-temporal
J7	median maxillary
J8	median palatine
D5	periodontal ligament
J9	temporo-mandibular joint
J10	mandibular symphysis (until fused)

AIR SPACES

A10	Maxillary sinus
A33	Mastoid air cells
A40	Nasal cavity
A50	Frontal sinus
A53	Sphenoid sinus
A70	Ethmoid air cells
A80	Pharynx

FISSURES, FORAMINA, AND DEPRESSIONS

F1	F. magnum
F2	F. ovale
F3	F. spinosum
F4	F. rotundum
F5	Mandibular foramen
F6	Mental foramen
F7	Lingual foramen
F8	Submandibular fossa
F9	Incisive foramen
F10	Greater palatine foramen
F11	Lesser palatine foramen
F12	Superior opening of lacrimal duct
F13	External auditory meatus
F14	Supra-orbital foramen
F15	Superior orbital fissure
F16	Optic foramen
F17	Inferior orbital fissure
F18	Infra-orbital foramen
F19	Zygomatic foramen
F20	Pterygo-maxillary fissure
F21	F. lacerum
F22	Grooves for meningeal vessels
F23	Grooves/canals for nutrient vessels, and miscellaneous neurovascular bundles

CANALS

C7   Inferior dental (alveolar) canal
C9   Nasopalatine canal
C12   Lacrimal duct
C23   Nutrient canals

SOFT TISSUES

S1   Tongue
S2   Lips
S3   Soft palate
S4   Gingiva
S5   Epiglottis
S6   Posterior pharyngeal wall
S7   Nose
S8   Ear lobes
S9   Eyes
S10   Eyelids

APPENDIX C
Examination of radiographs: checklist

BACKGROUND TO EXAMINATION

1. Patient profile: sex, age, racial or ethnic origin, home environment, diet, dental health care, etc.

2. Reason for taking the radiograph: patient's complaint.

3. Radiographic view: expectation of anatomical features that should be demonstrated.

4. Technical acceptability.

5. Correct viewing conditions:
   — quiet and concentration
   — dim room
   — bright white backlight and masking facilities
   — (magnifying glass)

DETAILED EXAMINATION

6. Symmetry.

7. Margins:
   — continuity
   — width

8. Bone consistency.

9. Dentition:
   — number of teeth
   — eruption status
   — morphology
   — condition

10. Supporting bone:
    — alveolar margins
    — periapical

11. Any other features:
    — radiolucent/radiopaque/combination
    — site
    — shape
    — size
    — margins
    — relation to other structures (?aetiological factors)
    — effect on other structures
    — provisional/differential diagnosis

12. Summary.

13. Proposals to meet patient's requirements, including other investigations.

RADIOLOGICAL SIEVE

- Normal
- Developmental
- Traumatic
- Inflammatory
- Cystic
- Neoplastic
- Osteodystrophy
- Metabolic/systemic
- Idiopathic
- Iatrogenic
- Foreign body
- Artefact

Appendix D
Specialized imaging techniques

In the course of investigating a patient's symptoms, there are a variety of imaging techniques that can now be employed. These are generally outside the scope of general dental practice, but a knowledge of the role they play in imaging the maxillo-facial region is nevertheless useful, to assist in deciding the most appropriate referral, and to help patients to understand special investigations that they may undergo.

The various techniques fall broadly into two categories: those using ionizing radiation and those using non-ionizing radiation. A brief description of the most commonly used techniques is provided in a common format, with sections on: energy source; pictorial display; mechanism; indications for use; advantages; and disadvantages.

1. *Ionizing radiation*

X-rays:
- Direct digital imaging
- Fluoroscopy
- Contrast examinations
— sialography
— TMJ (temporo-mandibular joint) arthrography
- Computed tomography (CT)

Radioisotopes:
- Nuclear medicine

2. *Non-ionizing radiation*

- Ultrasound
- Magnetic resonance imaging (MRI)

1. IONIZING RADIATION

X-rays

Direct digital imaging

Energy source: X-rays, from conventional machines. Digital (computer) images can be achieved by digitizing an existing radiographic film image, or creating direct digital images, without an intervening film stage. In direct digital imaging, the receptor is directly linked to a computer, resulting in real-time images being displayed on a visual display unit (VDU), or a special sensor is read by the computer. Direct digital systems are relatively common in general radiography, where there is a move towards *filmless* X-ray departments.

Pictorial display: black and white images on the VDU, which can be manipulated by purpose-designed software; the images can be printed out on thermal paper (Fig. D1).

Mechanism: a sensor is positioned in place of the film packet and exposed to X-rays, converting the X-ray signal into an electrical signal; the attenuation pattern detected is transferred to a PC (personal computer), where it is processed and the digital information converted into an analogue display. The sensor is re-usable, unlike film: two kinds of sensor are available at the present time. The first, and the most widely used, is connected to the computer by a fibre-optic cable, and is associated with instant images. The second is physically independent and has to be read by the computer, enabling sensors to be used at sites remote from the computer.

Indications for use: the technique can be used instead of conventional radiography.

Advantages: real-time images are particularly useful in endodontic therapy. The computer-stored images enable comparison of sequential images, allowing computer-assisted analysis to highlight subtle changes. A reduced exposure is

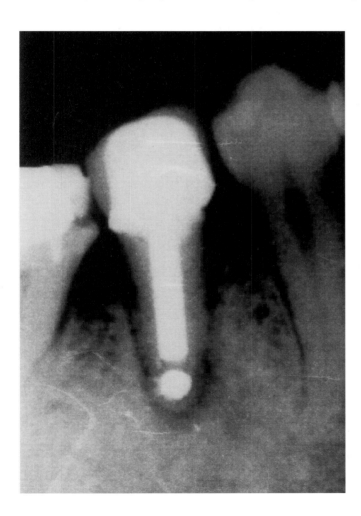

Fig. D1   Direct intra-oral digital image.

required to achieve individual images, when compared to conventional film radiography.

Disadvantages: cost — the acquisition of the hardware, software, sensor, print-out mechanism, and a suitable storage system represents a considerable capital outlay. The sensor area in most of the currently available models is less than that of an intra-oral film packet so that a full mouth examination would require a greater number of exposures, reducing the radiation dose benefit.

Fluoroscopy

Energy source: rotating anode X-ray tube, operating at a very low tube current, in the order of 1 mA (dental tubes operate at 7–15 mA; extra-oral units at 100 mA or more).

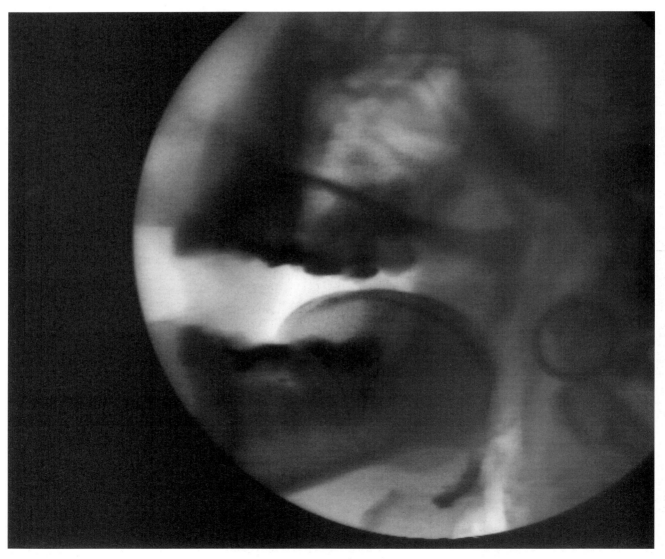

Fig. D2   Polaroid image from fluoroscopy examination of soft palate in speech: the black and white is reversed. The patient has velo-pharyngeal incompetency, and is unable to prevent nasal escape during speech: M 23.

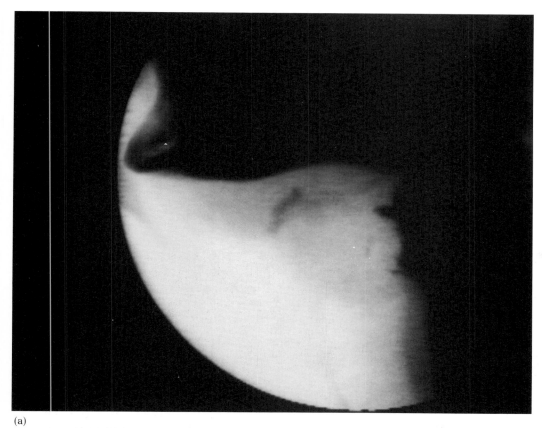

(a)

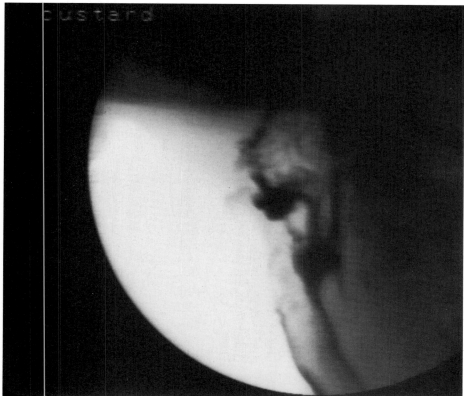

(b)

Fig. D3 Polaroid images from fluoroscopy
examinations of swallowing; the patients are
swallowing preparations containing barium.
(a) A normal swallow; the complete bolus is
passing into the oesophagus: M 23.
(b) Aspiration into the larynx and trachea: F 15.

Pictorial display: image portrayed in real time on VDU; can be recorded on videotape, or produce static polaroid images (Figs D2 and D3); concurrent X-ray images requiring a separate exposure, using conventional exposure factors, can also be made.

Mechanism: the X-ray beam is transmitted through the patient in the same way as in conventional X-ray imaging, the difference occurring primarily in the way in which the latent image in the X-ray beam is captured. An image intensifier replaces the conventional screen-film system, thus allowing a very low intensity beam to be used. The reduction in radiation dose that can be achieved enables continuous imaging to be carried out, to enable functional studies. Soft tissues are portrayed and can be enhanced by the use of barium-containing preparations.

Indications for use: in the head and neck region this technique is used for TMJ arthrography (see later section), and examination of speech and swallow disorders. Any invasive procedure requiring accurate imaging of moving structures is greatly assisted by fluoroscopy.

Advantages: low tube current enables increased time of exposure compared to conventional radiography. Speech examinations typically involve 15 to 60 seconds exposure time; swallow examinations approximately 1 to 3 minutes.

Disadvantages: equipment not normally available in dental centres due to high cost and relatively low demand.

Contrast examinations

Sialography

Energy source: X-rays. This technique is used to image the four major salivary glands (parotid and submandibular). It involves the introduction of iodine containing contrast medium, through the normal orifice, into the ductal system, and recording the filling of the ductal system on plain films; in some cases sialography is carried out in conjunction with computed tomography (CT).

Pictorial display: The ductal system is displayed on the radiographs as a radiopaque branching structure. It is normal to take two views, almost at right-angles in order to obtain a complete picture of the gland's relationships. Figures D4–D7 demonstrate some typical appearances.

Mechanism: the duct orifice is located and dilated; the duct is examined by introducing a lacrimal probe. The opening of the parotid duct (Stenson's duct) is in the buccal mucosa opposite the upper molars; the opening of the sub-mandibular gland duct (Wharton's duct) is in the floor of the mouth behind the lower incisors. Liquid contrast containing iodine is infused into the ductal system of the gland through the normal opening. 1–2 ml. of contrast is introduced through a plastic cannula, using hand pressure, hydrostatic pressure, or a pressure pump. Radiographs are taken to record an image of the ductal structure.

Indications for use: sialography provides information about the ductal structure of the salivary glands. Conditions in which this may be altered, or blocked, are particularly suitable for this investigation. The majority of patients present with swelling, often recurrent, which may or may not be painful. It is also a

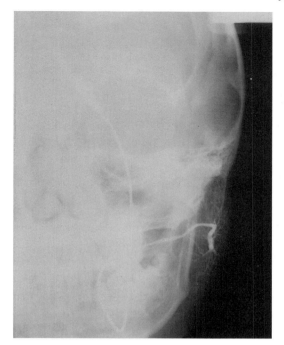
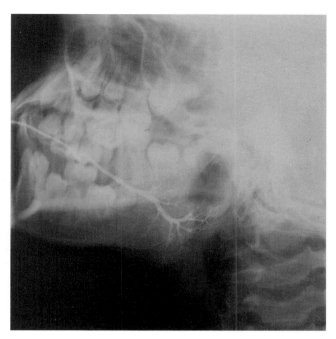

Fig. D4   Normal left parotid sialogram, AP and oblique lateral views; history of recurrent parotitis of childhood: M 11.

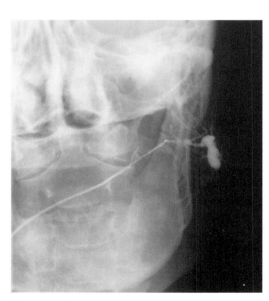
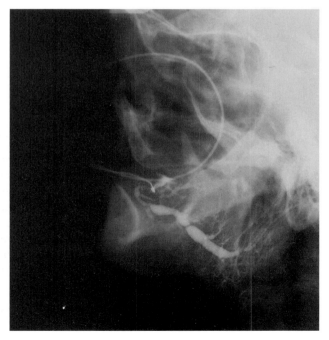

Fig. D5   Left parotid sialogram with evidence of dilatation and strictures, resulting from chronic inflammatory changes: M 72.

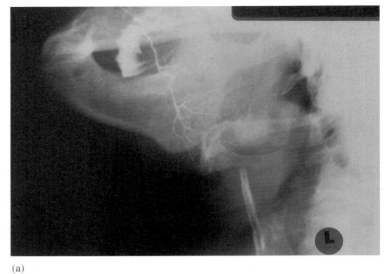

(a)

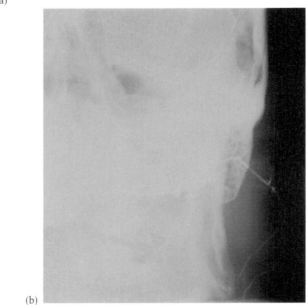

(b)

Fig. D6
(a) Normal appearance of parotid in oblique lateral view: M 45.
(b) Displacement of parotid gland in AP view, due to a malignant parotid tumour (same patient).

diagnostic tool for Sjögren's syndrome in which a typical radiologic appearance is seen (Fig. D7).

Advantages: sialography is one of the most straightforward ways to investigate salivary glands, and provides useful information about the ductal structure. The investigation is carried out in dental schools, as well as hospital radiology departments.

Disadvantages: only crude information about function can be obtained, if a clearing film is taken after a period of 10–20 minutes; this is much more accurately examined with a radioisotope investigation. The openings to the

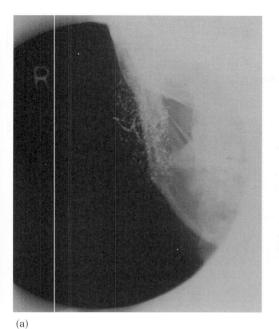
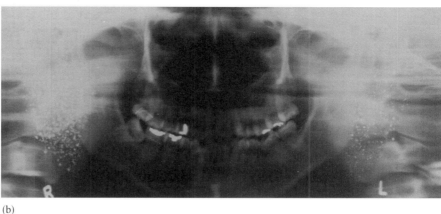

(a)   (b)

Fig. D7
(a) AP view of right parotid; typical punctate appearance seen in Sjögren's syndrome: F 26.
(b) Panoramic view; the left parotid sialogram was carried out a week previously using oil-based contrast. Function is severely reduced in Sjögren's Syndrome, causing a delay in clearing the contrast from the gland.

submandibular duct orifices are frequently extremely small, and may prove impossible to cannulate.

TMJ arthrography

Energy Source: X-rays, from conventional rotating anode tubes. Radiopaque contrast medium is injected into one or both of the TMJ (temporo-mandibular joint) spaces, in order to allow a judgement to be made about the disc position in both open and closed positions.

Pictorial display: the images are viewed real-time using fluoroscopy (see earlier section), and can be permanently captured on X-ray film (Fig. D8); separate exposures are necessary to create the two kinds of image.

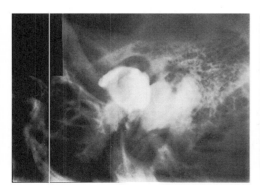
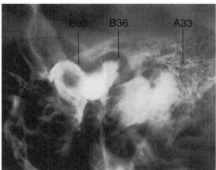
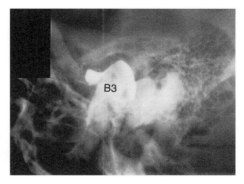

Fig. D8 Sequence of images in TMJ arthrography. (a) Closed position, normal appearance. (b) Open position, normal appearance. (c) Closed position with anterior displacement of disc altering the lower joint space. The anatomical features are identified with standard codes: F 40.

Mechanism: local anaesthetic infiltration is administered to the superficial tissues overlying the joint of interest; a hollow needle is then inserted, normally into the inferior joint space using the tactile information perceived through the needle in order to locate the head of the condyle; this and subsequent injection are carried out under fluoroscopic control; approximately 1 ml. of water-soluble iodine containing contrast is injected and the patient requested to open and close their mouth. The contrast is absorbed by the patient's own physiological mechanisms.

Advantages: the technique provides improved information about the disc status compared to plain film radiography.

Disadvantages: the disc itself is not demonstrated, and both compartments may inadvertently be injected, either due to a technical complication or as a result of perforations in the disc — the whole region is then opacified; the procedure can be very uncomfortable; the static images sent to the clinician contain only limited information. Improved information is obtainable by either arthroscopy or MRI.

Computed tomography (CT)

Computed tomography (CT) produces images of thin sections of the body on a VDU; the images are stored by computer, or on magnetic discs, and can be retrieved and manipulated; hard copy can be produced.

Energy source: X-ray tube, usually operating at 120 kVp, rotates 360 degrees around patient for each image section. Sensors detect the energy pattern in the attenuated beam at each circumferential point, transmit this to the computer in digital form for mathematical manipulation in order to produce a composite of the information relating to each section (slice) for storage and display.

Pictorial display: the stored digital information for each slice is converted into an analogue image portrayed on a VDU. The image includes all shades of grey between black and white. The extremes of black and white correlate with conventional X-ray images (Figs D9 and D10). Tissues each have a characteristic attenuation factor that can be ascribed a numerical value, using a scale first described by Hounsfield, and known as CT numbers, the range being from −1000 to +1000.

Characteristic CT numbers:

Air	−1000
Fat	−100 to −60
Water	0
Soft tissue	+40 to +60
Blood	+55 to +75
Dense bone	+1000

The displayed image can be manipulated by adjusting the *level* and the *window width*, according to CT numbers, to provide the most suitable image for the tissue type being investigated. A wide *window width* will include a large range of tissue types, but not demonstrate subtle changes; a narrow *window width* will demonstrate subtle change around the selected *level*. The final images on the VDU, or printed on film, include identification of the selected level and width.

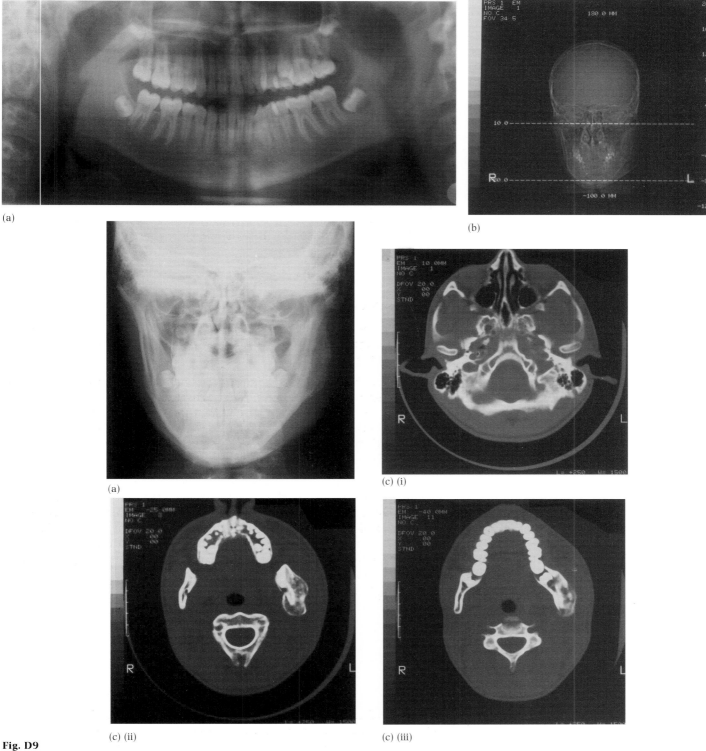

Fig. D9

(a) Conventional views demonstrate increase in size of left ramus: M 15.

(b) Scout (planning) view to show limit of scans.

(c) Axial CT images through the ramus; a diagnosis of osteomyelitis was made. (See Fig. 9.2 for further information.)

(i) Almost symmetrical image at level of condylar heads.

(ii) New bone visible on lateral and posterior aspects of left ramus; note the appearance of the ID canals.

(iii) New bone still evident at level of impacted third molars.

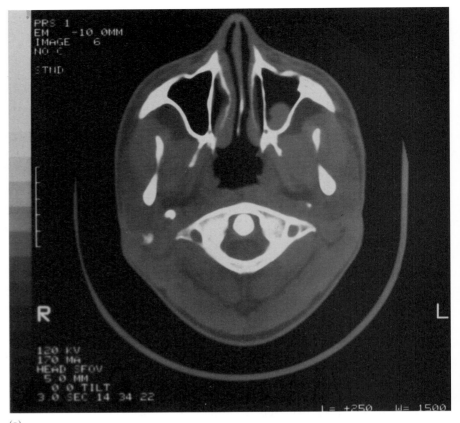

(a)

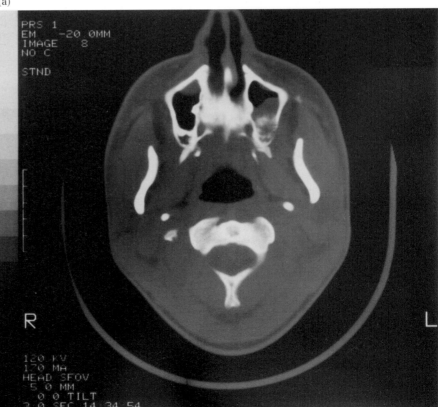

Fig. D10   Axial CT images through the maxilla in a
case of osteosarcoma: M 26. (See also Fig. 9.12.)
(a) Soft tissue present in left antrum; no change to
bone margins.
(b) There is erosion of the lateral wall of the antrum,
and mineralization within the lesion.

(b)

Mechanism: the patient is positioned on a table with the part of the body to be investigated within the central, circular, opening of a gantry; the patient's head and the gantry can be adjusted in order to image axial or coronal sections. Sagittal sections can be achieved on some patients but can also be generated by reformatting the stored images. Intravenous iodine-based contrast medium can be infused concurrently to demonstrate increased vascularity associated with pathology.

Indications for use: to determine the precise extent, and involvement of other structures, of soft and hard tissue tumours, severe infections, and extensive fractures of the middle third of the face; and in problematic diagnostic cases where conventional X-ray imaging has been inconclusive: in all these situations there is a need for high resolution sectional images to provide information that will assist in diagnosis and accurate treatment planning. The value of CT imaging in each case will be determined by the specialist investigating and treating the patient. CT scans are used by some specialists in assessing the available bone for the placement of implants; the cost and radiation dose to the patient must be carefully considered in such a situation, and balanced against the improved detail obtained compared with conventional radiographic techniques.

Advantages: high resolution, thin sectional images; good delineation of tissue interfaces; reformatting capability if continuous thin-section images are available in one plane (e.g. axial scans can be reformatted to produce coronal or sagittal sections).

Disadvantages: expensive; images not specific for tissue type; high radiation dose particularly if thin, overlapping slices: a typical plain skull film results in a dose to the patient in the order of 30 microsieverts (μSv), whereas a CT scan of the head results in a dose of approximately 4 millisieverts (mSv) (1000 microsieverts = 1 millisievert), giving in the order of 100 times greater dose; metallic objects cause streak artefacts which obscure information: fillings cause many problems with maxillo-facial imaging.

Radioisotopes

Nuclear medicine

Energy source: radioisotopes emitting gamma-rays at suitable levels for detection, and having a sufficiently short half-life to cause minimal risk to both the patient and others in their vicinity.

Pictorial display: real-time on a VDU after computer manipulation of acquired digital data; can be printed on X-ray film (Fig. D11).

Mechanism: the chosen radioisotope is linked to a suitable carrier for the medium being investigated, and injected intravenously; the medium is taken up by the tissues under investigation through physiological processes. The gamma-ray emissions are detected by a Na I (sodium iodide) scintillation crystal in a gamma camera, and the attenuation pattern analysed, stored, and displayed using computer systems.

Radioisotopes used for medical imaging:

Technetium (^{99m}Tc) — salivary glands, thyroid, blood, bone, liver, heart, lung

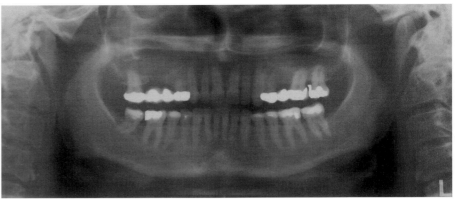

(a)

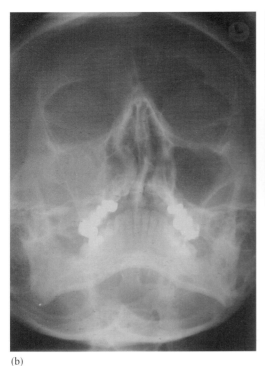

(b)

Fig. D11
(a) Loss of clear definition of the posterior wall of the right antrum in the panoramic view: F 54.
(b) Complete obliteration of the right antrum on the OM view, and destruction of the lateral wall. The lesion was diagnosed as adenocarcinoma.
(c) Technetium bone scan showing increased uptake in the right maxilla, due to tumour activity.

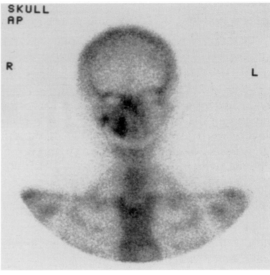

(c)

Gallium (^{67}Ga)   — tumours and inflammation
Iodine (^{123}I)   — thyroid
Krypton (^{81}Kr)   — lung

Technetium, with a half-life of 6 hours, is the most widely used radioisotope in the field of maxillo-facial imaging. It can be linked with the following carriers in order to ensure uptake in suitable organs:

In ionic form as pertechnetate (^{99m}TcO^{4-})   — salivary glands and thyroid
Methylene diphosphonate   — bone
Red blood cells   — blood
Sulphur colloid   — liver and spleen

Indications for use:
   ● Salivary gland function, as opposed to structure, for which sialography is ideal.
   ● Bone activity in cases of suspected metastases, continued condylar growth, infection.
   ● Assessment of breakdown of the blood–brain barrier.

Advantages: functional analysis is possible, particularly useful in salivary gland disorders such as Sjögren's syndrome, or atrophy; similar tissues throughout the body can be investigated with a single application.

Disadvantages: whole body radiation dose; lengthy investigation due to need to wait after introduction of radioisotope before imaging can begin; anatomical display of image is relatively poor.

2. NON-IONIZING RADIATION

Ultrasound

Energy source: ultra-high intensity sound, in the order of 1 to 15 MHz, produced by a piezo-electric transducer. Audible sound is in the range of 30 Hz to 16 000 Hz.

Pictorial display: the image is displayed real time on a VDU, and can be printed out on X-ray film or through polaroid systems (Fig. D12).

Mechanism: the ceramic transducer is activated by an applied voltage at the natural frequency of vibration of the ceramic; close contact is achieved between the transducer and the patient's skin by means of a gel and the beam of ultrasound directed at the region of interest. Tissue interfaces cause the sound to be reflected back, re-activating the transducer and resulting in an electrical voltage. The time delay between transmission and reception, and the strength of the received signal influence the analogue image displayed, and the ease with which tissue interfaces are detected.

Indications for use: investigation of soft tissue swellings, for example, tumours, infections, soft tissue cysts and salivary gland disorders; blood flow in vascular disorders.

Advantages: non-ionizing radiation that causes no adverse effects to human tissue. No limit on time of application, or repeat examinations.

Disadvantages: images are much less clear than those produced by X-ray techniques or MRI, and very dependent on the skill of the operator. Ultrasound can not travel through bone, therefore in practice, only soft tissue structures can be examined.

Magnetic resonance imaging (MRI)

Magnetic resonance imaging is often referred to as MRI, and sometimes as NMR imaging (nuclear magnetic resonance). It relies on the ability of certain elements of human tissue to respond to an applied magnetic field; hydrogen protons respond particularly well and are present in all tissues.

Energy source: a very powerful cylindrical magnet, in the order of 0.5 to 1.5 Teslas (T), and a radio frequency transmitter. To give an idea of the strength of such a field, it can be compared to the value of the the Earth's magnetic field at the surface of the Earth (0.6 gauss), and a fridge magnet (several hundred gauss).

10 000 (ten thousand) gauss = 1 Tesla.

Pictorial display: black and white sectional images are displayed on a VDU, in the same way as CT images are displayed; the allocation of black, white, and the range of greys is different to CT, and can be altered by the precise method

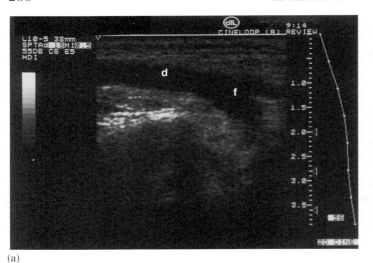

(a) (b)

Fig. D12
(a) Ultrasound examination of the left parotid salivary gland, in which the main duct (d) is dilated; the two branches at the fork (f) are also dilated: M 54.
(b) In a section transverse to the duct a large calculus (c) can be seen within the main duct.
(c) Sialography demonstrates the dilatation well; the calculus is difficult to detect as it has been surrounded by radiopaque contrast, and exhibits similar attenuation characteristics.

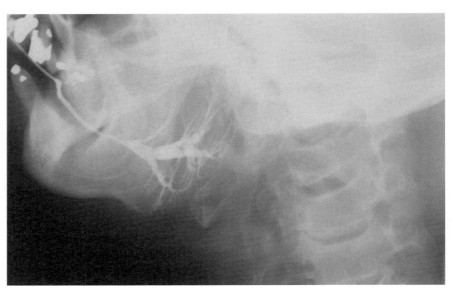

(c)

of acquisition of the information. The strength or weakness of the tissue emitted signal causes high signal and low signal areas in the images (Fig. D13).

Mechanism: The patient lies on a table inside a cylindrical tunnel which is formed by the core of the magnet. This is quite claustrophobic compared to the relatively open gantry of the CT machine. They are positioned in the centre of a strong magnetic field which causes the hydrogen nuclei to line up with the field. Application of a pulsed radio frequency causes these nuclei to spin, or *process*. When the radio frequency is switched off the protons relax and give off a signal themselves, in the form of another radio frequency — this is detected by a receiving antenna and analysed by computer to produce the displayed images.

Indications for use: assessment of intra-cranial and extra-cranial lesions, particularly involving soft tissue. The disc in the TMJ is shown, and the system is more tissue sensitive than CT.

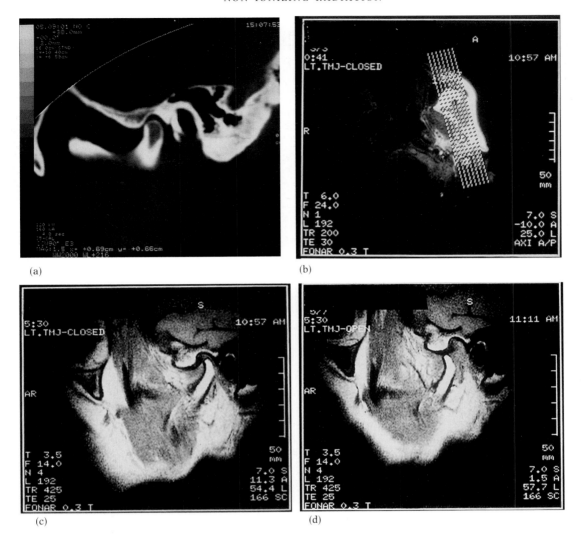

Fig. D13
(a) Sagittal CT scan through the TMJ — normal appearance: M 53.
(b) MRI scout view to show planned scans through the left TMJ: M 58.
(c) MRI scan, left TMJ — closed.
(d) MRI scan, left TMJ — open.
  Note the different black and white distribution of CT and MRI; cortical bone is seen as black in MRI due to its weak signal. The disc can be seen above the condylar head in the closed MRI view.

Advantages: the system does not use ionizing radiation, and there is little risk associated with application of magnetic fields to the majority of people. The exception to this is for those patients with artificial body parts which include magnetic materials (e.g. certain pacemakers). The sensitivity of the system is such that it can distinguish between different tissue types.

Disadvantages: cost; a suitable site in view of the weight of the magnet and the need to be remote from any metal equipment; claustrophobia induced by the tunnel; cortical bone is not imaged but depicted by the adjacent marrow and periosteum; patients with certain indwelling metal components cannot be imaged.

Bibliography

The following books, listed in alphabetical order by author, are recommended for further reading:

Roger Browne, Hugh Edmondson, and John Rout: *Atlas of Dental and Maxillofacial Radiology and Imaging.* Mosby-Wolfe.

Stephen Chapman and Richard Nakielny: *Aids to Radiological Differential Diagnosis.* Baillière Tindall.

Allan Farman, Christoffel Nortje, and Robert Wood: *Oral and Maxillofacial Diagnostic Imaging.* Mosby.

Paul Goaz and Stuart White: *Oral Radiology — Principles and Interpretation.* Mosby.

Stephen Porter and Crispian Scully: *Radiographic Interpretation of Orofacial Disease.* Oxford Medical Publications.

Eric Whaites: *Essentials of Dental Radiography and Radiology.* Churchill-Livingstone.

Index

abnormalities
  coronal and pericoronal   95–106
  morphological   57, 58 (*Fig.*)
  pulp and root   110–16
  see also artefact changes; cysts and
    cystic changes; developmental changes;
    iatrogenic changes; inflammatory
    changes; lesions; metabolic changes;
    radiolucencies; radiopacities; trauma
absorption, photoelectric   8–9
acidity   48, 104, 181
acute inflammatory change   127, 178
acute trauma   126, 176–83
adenocarcinoma   204 (*Fig.*)
aetiological factors   61–4
  inflammatory change   115
  short roots   116, 117
  trauma   176
age factors   **46**, 109, 115
air cavities/spaces
  anatomical features   37, 40, 188
  CT number   200
  maxillary sinus   39, 40, 51 (*Fig.*), 124–5
  periapical and periodontal   124
  radiolucency   59
aluminium filters   6, 29, 185
alveolar bone   38
ameloblastoma   64, 127, 144, 149–53 (*Figs*),
  157 (*Fig.*)
amelogenesis imperfecta   99 (*Fig.*), 103
anatomical features   18, 23–7 (*Figs*), **31–41**,
  186–9
  coding of   31–7, 186
  coronal and pericoronal   94–5
  location of   71
  periodontal/periapical   123
  pulp and root   108–110
  radiolucencies/radiopacities   122–5
  see also air cavities/spaces; bones
    and bony features; canals/channels; dental
    structures; depressions; fissures; foramina;
    jaws; joints; soft tissues; teeth
aneurysmal bone cysts   152 (*Fig.*)
angulation (of beam)   22
  horizontal angle   **19–21**, 80, 182–3
  right-angle   72–4, 196
  vertical angle   19–21, 182–3
  see also bisecting angle techniques

anode   **4**, 6, **184**, 194
antral septa   39
antrum (of Highmore), maxillary,   39
apices
  blood vessel damage   177
  open   46, 109, 113, 117
  see also periapical area
artefact changes
  coronal and pericoronal   106
  radiolucency   59, 142 (*Fig.*), **146**
  radiopacity   60, 61 (*Fig.*), **173**
atomic numbers   2, 6–9, 184, **185**
  bone   8, 59, 185
  cementum/dentine   38
  lead   5, 8 , 185
  soft tissue   8, 59, 185
  tungsten   4, 185
atom structure   6

barium   195 (*Fig.*), 196
basal bone   38
bimolar views   26–8
biopsy   67
bisecting angle techniques
  bitewings   19
  localization   80, 85–6, 90 (*Fig.*), 91
  occlusals   21
  periapicals   20, 23 (*Fig.*)
  periodontal disease   133
  radiolucencies   145 (*Fig.*)
  trauma   178 (*Fig.*), 181 (*Fig.*)
bitewings   19
  coronal/pericoronal changes   94 (*Fig.*)
  localization   71, 81–2
  periodontal disease   133
  radiolucencies   139 (*Fig.*), 150 (*Fig.*)
  radiopacities   168 (*Fig.*)
  symmetry   50, 51 (*Fig.*)
bone marrow   39
bones and bony features   33–6, 38–40,
  186–7
  absorption by   8
  atomic number   8, 59, 185
  cancellous   38, 39, 53, 62, 125
  computed tomography   200, 203
  consistency   53–4
  cortical   38, 39, 62, 64, 160

cysts   64, **142–3**, 149 (*Fig.*), 152–3 (*Figs*),
  157 (*Fig*)
  depressions   125
  loss   26 (*Fig.*), 132, 134–5 (*Figs*)
  margins   125
  mineral content   59–60
  nuclear medicine   203, 204
  Paget's disease of   115, 171 (*Fig.*)
  periapical and periodontal   122–36
  radiolucency/radiopacity   59
  resorption of   64
  Sharpey fibre   128
  Stafne cavity   61 (*Fig.*), 65, 71, 158
    (*Fig.*)
  trabeculae   38, 53–4, **125**
Bremsstrahlung radiation   7
BUILD acronym   78, 79 (*Fig.*), 80, 82
bulimia   48, 181

calcifications
  choroid plexus   164 (*Fig.*)
  lymph nodes   60, 87 (*Fig.*), 165 (*Fig.*)
  odontogenic cysts   **140**, 146 (*Fig.*), 148
    (*Fig.*)
  submandibular salivary gland   165 (*Fig.*)
  tonsils   162–3 (*Figs*)
calcium tungstate   14
calculus   133, 134 (*Fig.*), 206 (*Fig.*)
canals/channels   37, 40–1, 189
  inferior dental (alveolar)   40–1, 64
  multiple   110, 111 (*Fig.*)
  neurovascular   23 (*Fig.*), 124
  periapical and periodontal   124
  root   108, 110
cancellous bone   38, 39, 53, 62, 125
canine teeth   55
  chronological hypoplasia   165 (*Fig.*)
  impacted   88 (*Figs*)
  two-rooted   110, 111 (*Fig.*)
carcinomas
  adenocarcinoma   204 (*Fig.*)
  radiolucencies   147 (*Fig.*)
  radiopacities   166 (*Fig.*)
  squamous cell   155 (*Fig.*)
caries
  cervical   106
  deciduous teeth   102–3 (*Fig.*)

caries (*cont.*)
  dentine/enamel   52 (*Fig.*), 97 (*Fig.*), 102–3
    (*Fig.*)
  localization   70, 71
  pulpal vitality   126
  radiolucencies   104
  and sugar intake   48
cathode   4, 184
cemental dysplasia   133, 135 (*Fig.*), **136**, 142
    (*Fig.*), 157 (*Fig.*)
cementoblastoma   168 (*Fig.*)
cementoma   66 (*Fig.*)
cemento-osseous lesion   149–50 (*Figs*), 157
    (*Fig.*)
cementum   38, 108, 109, 113
centring points   19–22, 183
cephalometric views, *see* lateral cephalometric
    views
chemical damage   100 (*Fig.*), 104, **181**
children   26, 46
chronic inflammatory change   127–33, 197
    (*Fig.*)
chronic sclerosing osteomyelitis   162 (*Fig.*),
    170 (*Fig.*)
chronic trauma   126, 181
citrus fruit   48, 104, 181
cleft palate   139, 140 (*Fig.*)
clinical indications   48
  bitewings   19
  computed tomography   203
  direct digital imaging   193
  fluoroscopy   196
  lateral cephalometric view   29
  magnetic resonance imaging   206
  nuclear medicine   204
  oblique lateral view   28
  occipitomental projections   30–1
  occlusals   21, 22
  panoramic projections   23–6
  periapicals   19–20
  postero-anterior mandible projections   31
  sialography   196
  submentovertical projection   31
  ultrasound   205
coding of anatomical features   31–7, 186
collimator   5, 185
combination lesions
  examination of radiographs   **58–60**, 67
    (*Fig.*), 68
  lesions   160–73
combination techniques
  localization   72–4, 78–9 (*Figs*), **80–6**
Compton scatter   9
computed tomography (CT)   67, 200–3
  CT numbers   200
  radiolucencies   154 (*Fig.*)
  radiopacities   161 (*Fig.*), 169 (*Fig.*)
  and sialography   196

temporo-mandibular joint   207 (*Fig.*)
computer images, *see* computed tomography;
    resonance imaging; nuclear medicine
concrescence, root   113
condylar process   38
cone   5
connective tissue   38–9, 108
contrast radiography   86, 87 (*Fig.*), **196–200**,
    203
copper   4, 184
coronal and pericoronal changes   94–106
  fractures   176
  morphological   56–7, 58 (*Fig.*)
coronoid process   38
cortical bone   38, 39, 62, 64, 160
costs   194, 196, 203
cross-sectional radiographs
  inferior dental canal   41
  localization   72
  occlusals   **21–2**, 25 (*Fig.*), 27 (*Fig.*)
crowns, *see* coronal and pericoronal changes
CT scans, *see* computed tomography
cuspids   55
cysts and cystic changes   139–53
  bone   64, **142–3**, 149 (*Fig.*), 152–3 (*Figs*),
    157 (*Fig*)
  calcifying odontogenic   **140**, 146 (*Fig.*), 148
    (*Fig.*)
  coronal and pericoronal   104
  eruption   104, 105 (*Fig.*), **140**
  globulo-maxillary   148 (*Fig.*)
  localization   71
  mucous retention   60, 166 (*Fig.*)
  multiple jaw cysts   147 (*Fig.*)
  nasopalatine duct   142, 148 (*Fig.*)
  paradental   104, 105 (*Fig.*), **140**, 143 (*Fig.*)
  radiopacity   166
  soft tissue   205
  see also dentigerous cysts; keratocysts; radicu-
    lar cysts

deciduous teeth   54, 55, 102–3 (*Fig.*)
dens in dente   100
dental health care factors   46, 48
dental structures   32–3, 38, 186
  coronal and pericoronal   94–5
  examination of radiographs   63–4
  periapical and periodontal   122–5, 132
  pulp and root   108–10
  relationships between   70, 85
  thickness of   2, 60
  variation of   2, 9, 57
  see also anatomical features
denticle   98 (*Fig.*), 100
dentigerous cysts
  coronal/pericoronal changes   98 (*Fig.*), 104,
    105 (*Fig.*)

diagnosis of   64
localization   83 (*Fig.*)
radiolucency   **140**, 141 (*Fig.*), 143–5 (*Figs*),
    148 (*Fig.*)
radiopacity   167 (*Fig.*)
dentine   38, 108
  caries   97 (*Fig.*)
  dysplasia   114
  secondary   109, 115–16, 128 (*Fig.*), 181
    (*Fig.*)
  trauma   104
dentinogenesis imperfecta   113–14
dentition   54–7
  adult   19 (*Fig.*), 46
  deciduous   46, 54
  mixed   19 (*Fig.*), 46, 94 (*Fig.*)
  see also teeth
depressions   37, 125, 40, 188
developing and fixing   14–15
developmental changes   55–6
  arrest/cessation of   113, 118 (*Fig.*)
  coronal and pericoronal   94–104
  localization   71
  periapical   126
  pulp and root   108–14
  radiolucent lesions   139
  radiopaque lesions   164–5
  see also dysplastic conditions; hypoplasia
diagnosis   64–7
  computed tomography   203
  differential   65, 66 (*Fig.*), 140–57 (*Figs*),
    161–2 (*Figs*), 165–72 (*Figs*)
  ethnic factors   47
  incorrect   123
  neoplastic changes   71
  'radiological sieve'   **65**, **71**, 138, 160,
    191
  radiolucencies   139–58 (*Figs*)
  radiopacities   161–73 (*Figs*)
  see also examination of radiographs
dietary factors   46, 48
digital radiography   2, **192–4**, 200, 203
dilacerations   90–1, 110–11, 112 (*Fig.*)
dose of radiation
  high   203
  reduction of   13–14, 193–4, 196
  whole-body   205
double teeth   58 (*Fig.*), **99**, **111**, 113 (*Fig.*)
ductal system (of salivary glands) 196–8
dysplastic conditions
  cemental dysplasia   133, 135 (*Fig.*), **136**,
    142 (*Fig.*), 157 (*Fig.*)
  dentine dysplasia   114
  fibrous dysplasia   64, 71, 161 (*Fig.*), 170
    (*Figs*)
  odontodysplasia   99 (*Fig.*), 103, 114
  pulp and root changes   114
  see also developmental changes

elastic scatter   9
electrons   **7**, 9, 184
emulsion   10, 12, 13, **14**
enamel   38, 104
    caries   52 (*Fig.*), 97 (*Fig.*), 102–3 (*Fig.*)
    erosion   48, 181, 182 (*Fig.*)
    evaginations   57, 100
    invaginations   57, 58 (*Fig.*), 97 (*Fig.*), **100**, 111
    mineralization   103
    pearls   111, 112 (*Fig.*)
    pulp and root changes   115
    trauma   104
energy sources   3–7
    computed tomography   200
    direct digital imaging   192–3
    fluoroscopy   194
    magnetic resonance imaging   205
    nuclear medicine   203
    sialography   196
    TMJ arthrography   199
    ultrasound   205
environmental factors   46–8
eruption cysts   104, 105 (*Fig.*), **140**
ethnic factors   46, 47, 48 (*Fig.*)
evaginations   97 (*Fig.*), 100
examination of radiographs   44–68, 190–1
    and parallax principle   76
    strategy for   45, 49–50, 67–8
    see also diagnosis
exfoliation   130 (*Fig.*), 131–2
extra-oral projections   13–14, 18, 22–31, 73

fibroma   153 (*Fig.*), 157 (*Fig.*), 168 (*Fig.*), 170 (*Fig.*)
fibrous dysplasia   64, 71, 161 (*Fig.*), 170 (*Figs*)
film, X-ray   10–14, 19–20
    in specialized techniques   199, 200, 203, 205
filters, aluminium   6, 29, 185
fissures   37, 40, 188
fixing and developing   14–15
fluorescence   14
fluoridation   48
fluoroscopy   **194–6**, 199, 200
follicle   38, 141 (*Fig.*)
foramina   37, 40, 123–4, 188
foreign bodies
    localization   71
    radiolucency   146
    radiopacity   60, 172 (*Fig.*), 173
    trauma radiography   182
fractures   182
    coronal   176
    facial   203
    mandible   52 (*Fig.*)
    orientation of   71, 183

root   177, 178–9 (*Figs*), 182–3
functional studies   196, 198–9, 204–5

gadolinium   14
gallium   204
gamma-ray emissions   203
giant cell granuloma/lesion   64, 149–50 (*Figs*), 157 (*Fig.*)
glass envelope   4, 184
globulo-maxillary cyst   148 (*Fig.*)
granulomas   64, 129, 140–1 (*Fig.*), 149–50 (*Figs*), 157 (*Fig.*)
gutta percha   86, 87 (*Fig.*)

hard tissue   38–40
    radiolucency   138
    radiopacity   160
    tumours   203
    see also bone and bony features
head position   19–22
heat production/distribution   4–9
horizontal angles   **19–21**, 80, 182–3
hospital investigations   29
hypercementosis   115, 116 (*Fig.*)
hypomineralization   103
hypoplasia   57, 98 (*Fig.*), **103**, 106, 165 (*Fig.*)

iatrogenic changes
    coronal and pericoronal   106
    localization   71
    pulp and root   116
    radiolucent lesions   146
    radiopaque lesions   173
    trauma   178, 181
idiopathic changes
    localization   71
    osteosclerosis   66 (*Fig.*), 130, 172 (*Fig.*)
    pulp and root   116
    radiolucent lesions   146
    radiopaque lesions   167, 172 (*Fig.*)
imaging techniques
    radiographic, *see* radiographic images
    specialized   2, 67, **192–207**
incisor teeth   53, 56
    chronological hypoplasia   165 (*Fig.*)
    evaginations   100
    multiple canals   110, 111 (*Fig.*)
    peg-shaped   96 (*Fig.*)
    periapical cemental dysplasia   136
inelastic scatter   9
infection   127–8, 139, 140–1 (*Figs*)
    computed tomography   203
    nuclear medicine   204
    radiolucencies   146 (*Fig.*)

radiopacities   162 (*Figs*), 164 (*Fig.*)
    ultrasound   205
inferior dental canal   40–1, 64
inflammatory changes
    acute   127, 178
    chronic   127–32, 197 (*Fig.*)
    coronal and pericoronal   104
    localization   71
    and margins of lesion   63
    nuclear medicine   204
    periapical   **126–32**, 140 (*Fig.*), 178 (*Fig.*)
    periodontal   132–3
    pulp and root   115
    radiolucency   **139**, 141 (*Fig.*), 155 (*Fig.*)
    radiopacity   163 (*Fig.*), 165–6
    and resorption   64, 115
    and shape of lesion   62
    trauma   179 (*Fig.*)
information gathering   49–50, 65, 68 *see also* examination of radiographs
injury, *see* trauma
intra-oral projections   10–13, 18, 19–27, 82–5
invaginations   57, 58 (*Fig.*), 97–8 (*Figs*), **100**, 103, 111, 113 (*Fig.*), 180 (*Fig.*)
inverse square law   3, 5
iodine   196, 200, 203, 204
Ionising Radiations Regulations   3

jaws
    cysts   140, 147 (*Fig.*)
    lateral cephalometric views   28
    radiolucencies/radiopacities   39, 40
    see also mandible; maxilla
joints   36, 40, 188
    tempero-mandibular   196, **199–200**, 206–7
juvenile periodontitis   47, 134 (*Fig.*)

keratocysts
    coronal/pericoronal changes   104
    diagnosis   62
    radiolucency   **140**, 142 (*Fig*), 145–50 (*Figs*), 153 (*Fig.*), 157 (*Fig.*)
    radiopacity   166–7 (*Figs*)
krypton   204

lamina dura   128
lanthanum   14
lateral cephalometric view   28–30
    combined with others   72–3, 84 (*Fig.*)
    radiolucencies   147 (*Fig.*)
    radiopacities   164 (*Fig.*)
    symmetry   50–1
lateral oblique views   26–8, 29 (*Fig.*),
    radiolucency   141 (*Fig.*), 156 (*Fig.*)
    radiopacity   173 (*Fig.*), 197–8 (*Figs*)

lateral perforation   81
lead shielding   **4–5**, 8, 13, **184**
lesions
    benign   62–4, 71, **144**, 157 (*Fig.*), **166**, 168
        (*Figs*)
    cemento-osseous   149–50 (*Figs*), 157 (*Fig.*)
    combination   160–73
    cystic, *see* cysts and cystic changes
    description/features of   61–6
    extra-cranial   206
    giant-cell   64, 149–50 (*Figs*), 157 (*Fig.*)
    inflammatory, *see* inflammatory changes
    intra-cranial   206
    localization   70–92
    malignant   62–3, 64 (*Fig.*), 71, **144–5**, **166**,
        169 (*Fig.*), 198 (*Fig.*)
    neoplastic, *see* neoplastic lesions
    periapical/periodontal   61, 71
    radiolucent, *see* radiolucencies
    radiopaque, *see* radiopacities
    site of   61–2, 138, 160
    see also abnormalities; *names of individual*
        lesions and pathologies
Leung's premolar   97 (*Fig.*), 100
lighting conditions   49
localization issues   70–92
lymph node calcification   60, 87 (*Fig.*), 165
    (*Fig.*)

magnetic resonance imaging (MRI)   67, 205–7
magnifying glasses   49
mandible   33, 38–9, 186
    cross-sectional occlusals   21, 27 (*Fig.*)
    edentulous   52, 53 (*Fig.*)
    fractures   52 (*Fig.*)
    oblique lateral view   26, 28, 156 (*Fig.*)
    occlusal radiographs   21, **22**, 27 (*Fig.*)
    postero-anterior view, *see* postero-anterior
        mandible projection
    submandibular salivary gland   196, 199
    submentovertical view   31
    tempero-mandibular joint   196, **199–200**,
        206–7
margins   **51–3**, 54 (*Fig.*), 60 (*Fig.*), **63**, 64
    (*Fig.*), **125**
masking conditions   49
maxilla
    anatomical features   33, 39, 187
    computed tomography   202 (*Fig.*)
    cross-sectional occlusals   21
    occlusal radiographs   21, 22
    sinuses   39, 40, 51 (*Fig.*), 124–5
mesiodens   86 (*Fig.*), 89, 90
metabolic changes
    coronal and pericoronal   104–6
    localization issues   71
    pulp and root   115

radiolucent lesions   145–6
radiopacities   167
methylene diphosphonate   204
mineralization   59–60, 103
molar teeth   55
    bimolar views   26–8
    chronological hypoplasia   165 (*Fig.*)
    impacted   201 (*Fig.*)
    taurodontism   111
    three-rooted   110
mounting systems   15
mucous retention cyst   60, 166 (*Fig.*)
multiple myeloma   62, 156 (*Fig.*)
muscles, mandible   39
myeloma, multiple   62, 156 (*Fig.*)
myxoma   157 (*Fig.*)

nasopalatine duct cysts   142, 148 (*Fig.*)
neoplastic lesions
    benign   62–4, 71, **144**, 157 (*Fig.*), **166**, 168
        (*Figs*)
    computed tomography   203
    infected   162 (*Fig.*)
    localization   71
    malignant   62–3, 64 (*Fig.*), 71, **144–5**, **166**,
        169 (*Fig.*), 198 (*Fig.*)
    nuclear medicine   204
    radiolucencies   **144**, 149–52 (*Figs*), 154–6
        (*Figs*)
    radiopacities   162 (*Fig.*), 166
    ultrasound   205
neurovascular canals/channels   23 (*Fig.*), 124
nuclear medicine   203–5
nuclear magnetic resonance (NMR), *see*
        magnetic resonance imaging

oblique projections   21, 24–5 (*Figs*)
    combined with others   67 (*Fig.*), 80, 82–4
    lateral, *see* lateral oblique views
    localization   71, 86, 88–91
    radiolucencies   140 (*Fig.*), 142 (*Fig.*), 148
        (*Figs*), 154 (*Fig.*)
    trauma radiography   182–3
observation points   75–6
occipitomental projections   30–3
    radiolucencies   146 (*Fig.*)
    radiopacities   162 (*Fig.*), 167 (*Fig.*), 169–70
        (*Figs*)
    symmetry   51 (*Fig.*)
occlusal trauma   181
occlusals   21–2, 24–5 (*Figs*)
    cross-sectional, *see* cross-sectional radiographs
    localization   **82**, 83–5 (*Fig.*), 89, 90
    oblique, *see* oblique projections
    topographical   21
    'true', *see* 'true' occlusals

vertex   21–2, 25 (*Fig.*), 72–3, 86 (*Fig.*),
    92 (*Fig.*)
occlusal trauma   181
odontodysplasia   99 (*Fig.*), 103, 114
odontomes   98 (*Fig.*), **100–3**, 111, 113 (*Fig.*),
    168 (*Fig.*)
oil   5–6, 185
osteoclasts   64, 115, 130
osteodystrophies   71, 145, 167
osteitis
    rarefying   128, 130, 131 (*Fig.*), 141 (*Fig.*),
        181 (*Fig.*)
    sclerosing   60, 129–32, 172 (*Fig.*)
osteofibrosis   136
osteoma   168 (*Fig.*)
osteomyelitis   155 (*Fig.*), 161–2 (*Figs*), 170
    (*Fig.*), 201 (*Fig.*)
osteoporosis   54
osteosarcoma   161 (*Fig.*), 169 (*Fig.*), 202 (*Fig.*)
osteosclerosis   66 (*Fig.*), 130, 172 (*Fig.*)

Paget's disease   115, 171 (*Fig.*)
palate
    cleft   139, 140 (*Fig.*)
    soft   41, 194 (*Fig.*)
palatine process   39
panoramic projections   22–9
    combined with others   67 (*Fig.*), 73–4,
        80–6, 204 (*Fig.*)
    examining   44
    inferior dental canal   41
    intensifying screens   14
    localization   86 (*Fig.*), 88–92
    margin discontinuity   52, 53 (*Fig.*)
    patient movement   52, 53 (*Fig.*)
    periodontal disease   133
    radiolucencies   140–1 (*Figs*), 143–53 (*Figs*),
        155 (*Fig.*), 157–8 (*Figs*)
    radiopacities   161–3 (*Figs*), 165–72 (*Figs*)
    salivary glands   199 (*Fig.*)
    symmetry   50
    trauma   181 (*Fig.*)
paradental cysts   104, 105 (*Fig.*), **140**, 143
    (*Fig.*)
parallax   71, 74–80
    definition   75
    trauma   179 (*Fig.*), 181 (*Fig.*), 183
paralleling technique
    bitewings   133
    periapicals   **20**, 73, 80, 82, 85–6 (*Figs*),
        133, 178 (*Fig.*)
    periodontal disease   133
    trauma   178 (*Fig.*)
parotid gland
    calcification   163 (*Fig.*)
    sialography   196, 197–9 (*Figs*)
    ultrasound   206 (*Fig.*)

parotitis 197 (*Fig.*)
patient
  management, *see* treatment plans
  movement 52, 53 (*Fig.*)
  profiles 46–8
  sensitivity of 182
  understanding of techniques 193
periapical area 122–36
  cemental dysplasia 133, 136
  granuloma 129, 140–1 (*Fig.*)
  inflammatory change **126–32**, 140 (*Fig.*),
      178 (*Fig.*)
  lesions 61, 71
  localization issues 71, 87, 88 (*Fig.*), 91
  radicular cysts 129
  trauma **126**, 178–9 (*Figs*), 183
  X-rays **19–20**, 23–6 (*Figs*), 29 (*Fig.*), 41,
      80–1
pericoronal changes, *see* coronal and pericoronal
      changes
pericoronitis 104
periodontal disease 26 (*Fig.*), 122–36
  juvenile periodontitis 47, 134 (*Fig.*)
  localization 70, 71
periodontal ligament fibres/space 38
periodontium 126, 132
pertechnetate 204
phleboliths 87 (*Fig.*), 91
phosphorescence 14
photoelectric absorption 8–9
Pindborg tumour 146 (*Fig.*)
polaroid images/systems 194–6, 205
postero-anterior mandible projection 31, 34
      (*Fig.*)
  combined with other views 72, 73
  radiolucencies 147 (*Fig.*), 149 (*Fig.*), 152
      (*Fig.*), 155 (*Fig.*)
  radiopacities 161–3 (*Figs*)
premolar teeth 55
  evaginations 100
  hypoplasia/hypomineralization 103
  Leung's 97 (*Fig.*), 100
  two-rooted 110
processing of radiographs 2, 14–15
production of radiographs 2–16
pulp and pulp changes 38, 108–19
  chamber 38, 57, 108
  death 178
  stones 115
  trauma **114**, 176, 181
  vitality of 108, **126–7**, 177, 181

quality issues 48–9
  information gathering 49
  processing 15
  specialized techniques 205
  trauma radiography 182

racial factors 46, 47, 48 (*Fig.*)
radiation
  Bremsstrahlung 7
  characteristic 8
  dosage 13–14, 193–4, 196, 203, 205
  ionizing 3, 193–205
  leakage 4
  non-ionizing 205–7
  regulations 3
  white 7
  see also radiographic images
radicular cysts
  diagnosis of 63,
  periapical 129
  radiolucency **140–2**, 148–50 (*Figs*), 153
      (*Fig.*), 157 (*Fig.*)
  radiopacity 166 (*Fig.*)
radiographic images
  appearance, *see* radiographic projections
  contrast 86, 87 (*Fig.*), **196–200**, 203
  definition of 2
  developing and fixing 14–15
  digital 2, **192–4**, 200, 203
  displaying, *see* viewing systems
  enlargement of 49
  examination of 44–68, 76, 190–1
  high resolution 203
  identification of 15
  information from 49–50, 65, 68
  intensification of 13–14, 196
  interpretation of 44–68, 76, 190–1 *see also*
      diagnosis
  latent 14–15
  localization issues 70–92
  mounting of 15
  observation points 75–6 *see also*
      parallax
  permanent 14–15
  processing of 2, 14–15
  production of 2–16
  quality of, *see* quality issues
  real-time 193, 196, 199, 203, 205
  reasons for taking 44–5 *see also* clinical
      indications
  receptors 10–14
  regulations for 3
  retrievability of 15
  review of 66 (*Fig.*), 67
  scatter 8, 9
  sectional 203
  skills of operator 44, 205
  storage of 15
  summary of findings 65
  thoroughness in scrutinizing 68
  and vision 9–12
  see also atomic numbers; energy sources;
      radiation; radiolucencies; radiopacities;
      X-rays

radiographic projections 9–12, 18–31, 71–86
  bimolar views 26–8
  centring points 19–22, 183
  choice of 48, 182
  extra-oral 13–14, **18**, **22–31**, 73
  geometry 50–2, 72, 79 (*Fig.*), 85, 86 (*Fig.*),
      133
  head position 19–22
  intra-oral 10–13, 18–27, 82–5
  localization issues 70–92
  multiple 81, 83, 85, 182, 196 *see also*
      combination techniques
  see also angulation; bitewings; combination
      techniques; cross-sectional radiographs;
      lateral cephalometric views; oblique
      projections; occipitomental projections;
      occlusals; panoramic projections;
      parallax; paralleling technique;
      postero-anterior mandible projection
      submentovertical projection
radioisotope imaging 67, 203–5
'radiological sieve' **65**, **71**, 138, 160, **191**
radiolucencies **58–61**, 63, 65 **138–58**
  air cavities 59
  antral 39
  artefacts 59, 142 (*Fig.*), **146**
  bitewings 139 (*Fig.*), 150 (*Fig.*)
  bone 59
  carcinomas 147 (*Fig.*)
  caries 104
  cervical 106
  computed tomography 154 (*Fig.*)
  definition 58
  foreign bodies 146
  inflammatory changes **139**, 141 (*Fig.*), 155
      (*Fig.*)
  jaws 39, 40
  neoplastic lesions **144**, 149–52 (*Figs*),
      154–6 (*Figs*)
  periapical/periodontal 66, **122–5**, **128–30**,
      136, 140–57 (*Figs*)
  pulp 108
  soft tissue 59
  tooth germs 63 (*Fig.*), 95, 99, 139–40
      trauma 139
radiopacities **58–61**, 63, 66 (*Fig.*), **160–73**
  artefacts 60, 61 (*Fig.*), **173**
  bitewings 168 (*Fig.*)
  carcinomas 166 (*Fig.*)
  computed tomography 161 (*Fig.*), 169 (*Fig.*)
  definition 58
  foreign bodies 60, 172 (*Fig.*), **173**
  inflammatory change 163 (*Fig.*), 165–6
  jaws 39, 40
  localization 91, 92 (*Fig.*)
  neoplastic lesions 162 (*Fig.*), 166
  periapical and periodontal 122, **125**,
      129–30, 136, 167–8 (*Figs*)

radiopacities (*cont.*)
  pulp stones   115
  soft tissue   160
radiopaque markers   86–7, 199
Raleigh scatter   9
ramus   38
rare earth materials   14
rarefying osteitis   128, 130, 131 (*Fig.*), 141
      (*Fig.*), 181 (*Fig.*)
referral   192
regional odontodysplasia   103
roots   108–19
  additional   57
  bifid   58 (*Fig.*)
  canals   108, 110
  fractures   177, 178–9 (*Figs*), 182–3
  morphology   56–7, 110–11
  number of   110, 111 (*Fig.*)
  resorption   116, 119 (*Figs*), 127, **130–2**,
      179 (*Fig.*)
  shape abnormalities   57
  short   116–19, 130
  trauma   114, 176–83

salivary glands
  calcification   163 (*Fig.*), 165 (*Fig.*)
  nuclear medicine   203–5
  sialography   86, 165 (*Fig.*), **196–9**, 206
      (*Fig.*)
  ultrasound   205, 206 (*Fig.*)
scatter   8, 9
sclerosing osteitis   60, 129–32, 172 (*Fig.*)
sclerosing osteomyelitis   162 (*Fig.*), 170 (*Fig.*)
screens, intensifying   13–14
self-assessment examples   91–2
sex factors   46, 47, 110
Sharpey fibre bone   128
sialography   86, 165 (*Fig.*), **196–9**, 206 (*Fig.*)
silica   184
silver bromide   12, 14, 15
sinuses   39, 40, 51, 86, 124–5
Sjögren's syndrome   198, 199 (*Fig.*), 205
skills of radiography   44, 205
skull   31, 35 (*Fig.*), 156 (*Fig.*)
SLOB acronym   76, 78, 82
socio-educational factors   47
soft drinks   48, 104, 181
soft palate   41, 194 (*Fig.*)
soft tissue
  absorption by   8
  air in   59
  anatomical features   37–9, 41, 189
  atomic number   8, 59, 185
  calcium in   163 (*Fig.*)
  CT number   200
  cysts   205
  fluoroscopy   196

lateral cephalometric views   29
magnetic resonance imaging   206
  radiolucency   59
  radiopacity   160
  trauma   182
  tumours   203
  ultrasound   205
solitary bone cysts   64, 142 (*Fig.*), 149 (*Fig.*),
      153 (*Fig.*), 157 (*Fig*)
solitary plasmacytoma   62
speech disorders   196
squamous cell carcinoma   155 (*Fig.*)
Stafne cavity   61 (*Fig.*), 65, 71, 158 (*Fig.*)
Stenson's duct   196
storage systems   2, 15
submandibular salivary gland   196, 199
submentovertical projections   **31**, 35 (*Fig.*), 72
sugar and dental caries   48
sulphur colloid   204
supernumerary teeth   55, 56 (*Fig.*), 63 (*Fig.*),
      100
  ethnic factors   47, 48 (*Fig.*)
  localization   71, 80–5, 89–92
  multiple   97 (*Fig.*)
  radiolucencies   140 (*Fig.*)
sutures   36, 40, 188
swallowing
  fluoroscopy techniques   195–6
  teeth   180 (*Fig.*)
symmetry   50–1

talon cusp   97 (*Fig.*), 100
taurodontism   110–12
technetium   203, 204
teeth
  apices   46, 109, 113, 117, 177 *see also*
      periapical area
  avulsed   177, 179 (*Figs*)
  condition of   57
  congenitally absent   55–7, 98 (*Fig.*)
  crown of, *see* coronal and pericoronal changes
  deciduous   54, **55**, 102–3 (*Fig.*)
  development sequence   55
  dilacerated   90–1, 110–11, 112 (*Fig.*)
  displacement of   64, 177, 180–1 (*Figs*)
  double   58 (*Fig.*), **99**, **111**, 113 (*Fig.*)
  ectopic   101 (*Fig.*), 103
  eruption status   56, 114
  form of   95, 99–103
  fusion of   99, 110, 111, 113
  gemination   98 (*Fig.*), 99, 110, 111
  germ   63 (*Fig.*), 95, 111, 139
  hypoplastic, *see* hypoplasia
  inhaled   177
  injury to, *see* trauma
  invaginated, *see* invaginations
  migration of   62, 101 (*Fig.*), 103, 104

morphology   56–7
number of   54–6
permanent   54, 55
position of   99, 103–4
pressure on   126, 127, 182
resorption of   64, 104, 115, 127
size of   96 (*Figs*), 99
structure of   38
subluxation   177–8, 180 (*Fig.*)
submerging   101 (*Fig.*), 104
supplemental   56 (*Fig.*), 97 (*Fig.*), **100**, 139
      (*Fig.*)
swallowed   180 (*Fig.*)
taurodont   110–12
tenderness   127
toothbrush abrasion of   181 (*Fig.*)
transposition of   100 (*Fig.*), 103
transverse   101 (*Fig.*)
Turner tooth   98 (*Fig.*), 103
unerupted   71, 114
within teeth   100
see also canine teeth; dentition;
      incisor teeth; molar teeth; premolar teeth;
      pulp and pulp changes; roots;
      supernumerary teeth
tempero-mandibular joint (TMJ)   196,
      199–200, 206–7
tissue/s
  attenuation factors   200
  connective   38–9, 108
  variation of   2, 9
  see also hard tissue; soft tissue
TMJ, *see* tempero-mandibular joint
tongue   41
tonsillar calcifications   162–3 (*Figs*)
topographical occlusals   21
tori   125, 161 (*Fig.*)
trabeculae   38, 53–4, **125**
trauma   176–83
  acute   126, 176–83
  chemical   100 (*Fig.*), 104, **181**
  chronic   126, 181
  coronal and pericoronal   104
  late recognition of effects   183
  localization   71
  periapical   **126**, 178–9 (*Figs*), 183
  physical   176–7, 181
  pulp/root   114, 176–83
  radiolucent lesions   139
  see also foreign bodies
treatment plans   45, 64–6, 71, 203
'true' occlusals   21–2
  localization   72–4, 79–80 (*Figs*)
  radiolucencies   144–5 (*Figs*), 150–2 (*Figs*),
      157 (*Figs*)
  radiopacities   168 (*Fig.*)
tube, X-ray   3–5, 184–5
  anode   **4**, 6, **184**, 194

cathode **4**, 184
position changes   76, 80, 82, 87
see also angulation
tumours
  hard/soft tissue   203
  Pindborg   146 (*Fig.*)
  see also neoplastic lesions
tungsten   4, 6, 7, 184
Turner tooth   98 (*Fig.*), 103

ultrasound   67, **205**, 206 (*Fig.*)

vertex occlusals   21–2, 25 (*Fig.*), 72–3, 86
      (*Fig.*), 92 (*Fig.*)
vertical angles   19–21, 182–3
videotape   196
viewing systems   15–16, 49, 71–2
  computed tomography   200
  direct digital imaging   193
  fluoroscopy   196

magnetic resonance imaging   205–6
nuclear medicine   203
sialography   196
TMJ arthrography   199
ultrasound   205
views, *see* radiographic projections
vision and radiography   9–12
visual display units (VDUs)   192–3, 196, 200,
      203, 205
vitality, pulpal   **126–7**, 177, 181
voltage   4, 7, 8

water
  CT number   200
  fluoridation   48
Wharton's duct   196
white radiation   7
window   5, 200

X-rays   192–203

beams   5–8, 183, 196
damage caused by   3
distance from skin   5
dosage, *see* dose of radiation
film, *see* film, X-ray
filmless, *see* digital radiography
interaction with matter   7–9
leakage of   4
low-energy/intensity   6, 196
photons   7, 8, 9
properties of   3
source of, *see* energy sources
tube, *see* tube, X-ray
see also radiographic images
Y-line of Ennis   23 (*Fig.*), 39

zygomatic arches   31
zygomatic process   39, 125